HIV/AIDS and the Older Adult

HIV/AIDS and the Older Adult

Edited by
Kathleen M. Nokes
City University of New York, Hunter College
Hunter-Bellevue School of Nursing
New York, New York

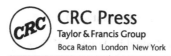

CRC Press
Taylor & Francis Group
Boca Raton London New York

CRC Press is an imprint of the
Taylor & Francis Group, an **informa** business
A TAYLOR & FRANCIS BOOK

HIV/AIDS AND THE OLDER ADULT

First published 1996 by Taylor & Francis

Published 2023 by CRC Press
Taylor & Francis Group
6000 Broken Sound Parkway NW, Suite 300
Boca Raton, FL 33487-2742

ISBN 13: 978-1-56032-430-0 (pbk)

Visit the Taylor & Francis Web site at
http://www.taylorandfrancis.com

and the CRC Press Web site at
http://www.crcpress.com

This book was set in Times Roman by Sandra F. Watts. The editors were Christine Williams and Kathleen P. Baker. Cover design by Michelle Fleitz. Printing and binding by Braun-Brumfield, Inc.

A CIP catalog record for this book is available from the British Library.

Library of Congress Cataloging-in-Publication Data

HIV/AIDS and the older adult / edited by Kathleen M. Nokes.
    p. cm.
  Includes bibliographical references.

    1. AIDS (Disease) in old age. 1. Nokes, Kathleen M. (Kathleen Mary)
RC607.A26H557 1996
362.1'989769792—dc20   95-41714
                                                         CIP

To older persons who are both infected and affected by HIV/AIDS

Contents

Foreword

It's as if the AIDS virus had been designed to exploit every gap in our scientific knowledge, every fault line in our social systems, every sad historical heritage of discrimination and distrust. Fund medical research to learn almost exclusively about how diseases develop (and largely neglect the study of the body's response to these same diseases), and we start the second decade of the global AIDS epidemic with a very imperfect understanding of the workings of the immune system. Construct a society so that there are gross inequities of wealth, and we yield sizable populations who engage in risk-taking behaviors for HIV infection, if only as a means of getting through life. Conduct "scientific research" on the epidemiology of a sexually transmitted disease among African American men that violates basic precepts of medical ethics (the Tuskegee syphilis study), and we yield a community at elevated risk of HIV infection that has good reason to distrust the public health and medical establishments when it comes to dealing with STDs. Treat gay men so that they are raised to believe that the worst thing that they could possibly be is who they actually are, and we yield populations whose very lives depend on sexual safety when they are loved—sometimes for the very first time—for the very quality that evokes hatred and fear almost everywhere else in their lives. Respond to an epidemic of drug abuse with a "war on drugs" rather than by dealing with the causes of drug abuse and devising effective medical treatments for addicts, and we yield a situation in which interventions that have been demonstrated to prevent AIDS among injecting drug users and their sexual partners become politically impossible to implement. Disparage behavioral researchers who attempt to learn more about the sexual lives of humans (and refuse to fund their research), and we begin yet another serious sexually-transmitted disease epidemic of the late 20th century by relying on sex behavior data provided by a courageous pioneer nearly a half-century earlier. Perhaps our political leaders should feel honored by the fact that so many people who live in risk of contracting AIDS believe that a virus of such lethal consequences, so adept in its ability to use human frailties and societal injustice as a vehicle for propagation, could actually be the result of government work.

Against this depressing background, it should come as no surprise that we don't know enough about the AIDS epidemic among people past the age of 50. Nor should it shock the reader that most Americans remain unaware of the fact that approximately 10% of the AIDS epidemic is diagnosed among people aged 50+ and that we may well pass the sad benchmark of having logged more AIDS diagnoses among older Americans than American deaths incurred during the Vietnam war. We have yet to see any focused effort to prevent new HIV infections among people aged 50+, nor do we have anything past a handful of media stories in the way of a public acknowledgment that the epidemic is not found only among the young.

It is obvious that the time has come to face the dangers posed by the AIDS epidemic, in part by learning more about how late middle-aged and older Americans are reacting to the epidemic. This book sets out to explore many aspects of this epidemic while also revealing and identifying gaps in service to older people with HIV/AIDS. We would like to highlight some central research agendas that we believe should be addressed if we are to do a better job of preventing and treating AIDS among Americans past the age of 50, and helping them to cope with the many other ways that the AIDS epidemic may affect them. We would like to start this list by outlining what is known about the epidemic among Americans past the age of 50.

Late middle age and old age are generally regarded among Americans as a time of decreasing sexual activity, to the point that we sometimes treat our elders as sexless or, even worse, as the object of crude or patronizing jokes when an interest in sex is evident among adults past a certain age. And indeed, national survey data collaborate this general perception *to a point*: prevalence rates of current celibacy increase with age and the proportion of the population that is sexually-risky declines with increasing age. In contrast to these general trends, however, is the fact that risky heterosexual adults past the age of 50 are substantially less likely to use condoms or undergo HIV testing than are adults in their 20s who are taking the exact same behavior risks for HIV transmission. Whether these patterns among older risk-takers are the result of the prevailing stereotypes of low sexual activity among the middle-aged and older (and hence perceived low risk for HIV) remains an open question.

Thus, one of the first questions that must be addressed if we are to do a better job of preventing new HIV infections among middle-aged or older adults is to understand more about seniors who are sexually risky. What are the corre-lates of sexual risk-taking within this age group? Do we need to try special methods to reach older homosexually-active men for prevention purposes? What are the best ways to reach risky older heterosexual adults? What kinds of inter-ventions would seem to be most effective for this group? Is it possible to con-struct a theory of risk-taking for HIV infection that holds relevance across the life course, or should understandings of risk-taking be specific to particular stages of the life course? None of these questions have been answered, yet they are central to the design of prevention programs specific to the needs of older Americans.

A second set of questions have to do with the care of older individuals with HIV infection. How do Americans past the age of 50 experience an AIDS diagnosis? Do our care systems operate so that older persons with HIV are, de facto, excluded from accessing services? How do older persons with AIDS ac-cess the informal care support systems that gay men with AIDS report as being so useful to their ability to cope with the effects of HIV disease? Do older persons with AIDS have needs that are specific to their age, or can generalized care services be provided irrespective of age? Are older Americans with HIV infection diagnosed in time for them to consider early intervention strategies, or does diagnosis generally occur after a serious opportunistic infection? Are there special drug adherence issues to consider that may be especially important among Americans past the age of 50? The health care and medical needs of older people with HIV/AIDS are examined in this book. There are also chapters de-voted to long-term care and the development of support groups. These are cru-cial to the quality of life for people living with HIV/AIDS.

It should be obvious by now that the AIDS epidemic affects people who remain uninfected with HIV, and even those who not are at any special risk of infection. Growing numbers of American cities and communities contain too many citizens who are too familiar with the duties of AIDS caregiving, of the rituals of death and the cycles of bereavement. Little is now known of the ability of older Americans to offer care to persons dying of AIDS, other than this ability seems to vary enormously across individuals. How do older parents deal with the news of an AIDS diagnosis among younger kin or friends, particu-larly when this announcement often contains within it the subtextual announce-ment of participation in nontraditional sexual behavior or drug use? To what extent do the health problems of older Americans themselves prevent them from being able to care for younger persons with AIDS? If there are grandchildren, do grandparents tend to become "parents" again and how do grandparents and grandchildren cope with this unexpected change in their relationship? Chapters within this text are devoted to these caregiving issues. Caregivers need a lot of support to navigate the process of helping someone else cope with a painful and fatal illness. Do older Americans find needed support within their friendship/kin networks to care for others when the illness in question is AIDS? Does the caregiving/grieving process harm the health of older people who provide help to those who are dying of AIDS? How do older parents cope after their children die of AIDS? Readers will find detailed descriptions of support groups and networks in this work.

It has been six years since the first book on the effects of AIDS among older Americans was published (Riley & Zablotsky, 1989).[1] It is gratifying to see that the work begun by the groundbreaking editors and authors of that book continues in *HIV/AIDS and the Older Adult.* This book makes strides in identifying the isolation of older people living with HIV/AIDS. We hope that this research tradition will continue until such time that the questions briefly outlined in this foreword—and in the remainder of this book—are adequately addressed, not only for Americans past the age of 50, but for all of us who are living with the repercussions of this awesome global epidemic.

Ron Stall and Joe Catania
Center for AIDS Prevention Studies
University of California
San Francisco

---

[1]Riley, M., & Zablotsky, D. (1989). *AIDS in an Aging Society: What We Need to Know.* New York: Springer Publishing Co.

Preface

Although the issue of HIV/AIDS in an older population is increasingly being recognized, it still remains a neglected area of focus. The current volume brings together clinicians who have cared for older persons with HIV/AIDS and provides an opportunity to share their experiences in the hope that their successes can be replicated and their stumblings avoided.

In chapter 1, Puleo describes the scope of the HIV epidemic, with special emphasis on its incidence in older populations. On the basis of the current lack of inclusion of older clients in HIV primary prevention strategies, she predicts that the virus will continue to spread unchecked in this population.

In chapter 2, the health care needs of persons with HIV/AIDS are described and an overview of the pathophysiology of HIV disease in older clients is presented. Primary, secondary, and tertiary prevention strategies form the organizing framework for this chapter. The comorbidity of tuberculosis and HIV disease in older clients is discussed.

Aupperle addresses the medical needs of persons with HIV/AIDS in chapter 3. The controversy surrounding the prognosis of older persons with AIDS as compared with that of younger persons with AIDS is explored. AIDS dementia is differentiated from the neurological manifestations of Alzheimer's disease.

Psychosocial issues are explored by Solomon in chapter 4. She addresses how the client's belief system affects interactions with health care providers. Through her interactions with older persons with HIV/AIDS, she has been struck by the degree of secrecy and isolation that characterizes many of these people's lives.

In chapter 5, Kornhaber and Malone describe how they created a support group for older persons with HIV/AIDS within a tertiary care facility. They review the process of establishing a need for the group and share how they have worked together as cofacilitators. Feedback from the group sessions is used to identify common themes.

Anderson addresses issues specific to older gay men and HIV/AIDS in chapter 6. He describes how Senior Action in a Gay Environment responded to the identified needs of their clients and developed an AIDS-specific intervention. Case examples are used to identify a variety of issues common to this population.

Wyatt presents the dilemmas of long-term care for older persons with AIDS in chapter 7. Home care and other housing issues are explored along with a discussion of nursing homes for persons with HIV/AIDS. Hospice care for those in the last stage of life is also presented.

In chapter 8, Carver and Brown explore the legal and ethical issues that older persons with HIV/AIDS face. They address employment protection for those who are still able to work. Elder abuse is explored, with special emphasis on the unique issues of older persons with HIV/AIDS who may be reluctant to reveal a "taboo" relationship. Planning for incapacity through implementation of advance directives is described in depth.

Caregiver issues are addressed in chapter 9 by Levine-Perkell. She explores special challenges experienced by caregivers of aged persons with HIV/AIDS, elderly parents who are caregivers to their children with HIV/AIDS, and grandparents raising grandchildren orphaned by the epidemic.

Joslin and Nazon describe in chapter 10 a variety of formal AIDS and aging networks that have been established throughout the United States. A rationale for establishing these networks is presented along with three case examples: New York, Florida, and New Jersey. The challenges, benefits, and organizational needs of building and maintaining these networks are explored.

Chapter 11 presents the voices of health and social service providers working in the AIDS and aging field and with older persons living with HIV/AIDS. Interviews were conducted with people throughout the United States to avoid a narrow regional perspective. Hickey provides a vehicle for these frontline providers and clients to share their stories. It is these voices that continue to motivate to action.

This book is directed toward health (nurses, physicians, physician assistants, gerontologists) and social service (social workers, psychologists, counselors, and case managers) providers of care for older persons with HIV/AIDS. Although it is not meant to be a piece of research, it does identify gaps in service and the almost overwhelming isolation of older persons with HIV/AIDS. The purpose of the book is to describe the experiences of people who have been working in the field, collaborating and sharing resources.

The HIV/AIDS and Aging Task Force of New York City, organized by the

Brookdale Center on Aging at the City University of New York, Hunter College (described in Chapter 10), was approached by Elaine Pirrone of Taylor & Francis about preparing a book because of its groundbreaking work in heightening awareness of HIV/AIDS in older populations. Members of this task force contributed a number of chapters, and the Education Committee of the task force participated in its ongoing development. Ms. Pirrone continued her active involvement throughout the entire project, and for that we are very grateful. In addition, the editor would like to thank Joanne Puleo for her assistance during the early stages of the project and Mark Bibbins for his expert editing of the chapters.

It has been more than 6 years since Riley, Ory, and Zablotsky[1] stated that "the place of older persons in the AIDS epidemic can no longer be overlooked" (p. 216). It is hoped that this volume will add a human dimension to the face of HIV/AIDS in the older population and convince the public and the policymakers that HIV/AIDS in older people cannot continue to be ignored.

Kathleen M. Nokes
City University of New York, Hunter College
Hunter-Bellevue School of Nursing

---

[1]In *AIDS in an Aging Society: What We Need to Know*, published in 1989 by Springer.

Contributors

Gregory Anderson, M.S.W., C.S.W., has done considerable work in the field of gay and lesbian gerontology. As Supervisor of Individual Services at Senior Action in a Gay Environment, he was instrumental in implementing a comprehensive social service program for older gay men with HIV/AIDS. He is a former co-chair of the HIV/AIDS and Aging Task Force of New York and is a 1995 Diego Lopez AIDS Service Award recipient for his contribution to social work in the field of HIV/AIDS. He is currently HIV Patient Coordinator for Schenectady Family Health Services in Schenectady, New York.

Peter Aupperle, M.D., M.P.H., is an Assistant Professor of Psychiatry at the Albert Einstein College of Medicine in New York City. He is Board Certified in both general and geriatric psychiatry, and is Chief of the Geriatric Psychiatry Clinic at Hillside Hospital, Long Island Jewish Medical Center. Dr. Aupperle is a member of the HIV/AIDS and Aging Task Force at the Brookdale Center, Hunter College, as well as a consultant to the AIDS Mental Hygiene Project at the School of Education, New York University. He has presented on the topic of AIDS and the Elderly at several national gerontological and psychiatric meetings.

A. Widney Brown, J.D., is the HIV-Related Violence Program Coordinator at the New York City Gay and Lesbian Anti-Violence Project. She provides legal service to HIV-positive victims of violence.

Joe Catania, Ph.D., is an Associate Professor in the Department of Behavioral Medicine at the University of California, San Francisco. He is currently directing a series of large-scale national studies to elucidate the epidemiology of AIDS.

Kathleen Carver, R.N., M.A., J.D., is the Director of Legal Affairs at Village Center for Care in New York City, which operates home care, day treatment, and residential health care programs for people living with HIV. Prior to becoming an attorney, she was an educator and clinical nurse specialist in HIV.

Dorothy E. Hickey, M.A., M.P.H., R.N., C, is a Clinical Nurse Specialist who works with aging people in a Naturally Occurring Retirement Community in New York City. Her professional expertise is in community mental health and gerontology with a special interest in group work. She is a GEC Associate of the Brookdale Center on Aging and active in the State Society on Aging of New York.

Daphne Joslin, Ph.D., M.P.H., is an Assistant Professor in the Department of Community Health at the William Paterson College of New Jersey where she also serves as Coordinator of the Gerontology Program. She is a member of the New York City HIV/AIDS and Aging Task Force and is co-chair of the HIV/AIDS and the Elderly Workgroup of the Coalition on AIDS in Passaic County (CAPCO) New Jersey. Dr. Joslin is co-author with Anne Brouard, M.D., of the article "The Prevalence of Grandmothers as Primary Caregivers in a Poor Pediatric Population," which reports on their study of grandparents in New York City who are raising children orphaned by the epidemic.

Barbara Kornhaber, M.S., R.N., B.S., is the Needlestick Coordinator at Mt. Sinai Medical Center in New York. She evaluates, counsels, and intervenes with all exposed and source contacts in each blood/body fluid exposure incident. Ms. Kornhaber is also co-founder and co-facilitator of a Support/Education Group for HIV/AIDS people over the age of fifty. She is a member of the HIV/AIDS and Aging Task Force and one of two designated trainers selected by the NYSDOH-AIDS Institute to train counselors for HIV Antibody Pre- and Post-Test Counseling.

Joan Levine-Perkell, M.S.W., A.C.S.W., is a clinical social worker in the Geriatric Psychiatry Clinic at Hillside Hospital, Long Island Jewish Medical Center in New York, where she provides individual, couple, and group psychotherapy. She is also a certified HIV/AIDS counselor and trainer, co-chair of the Brookdale Center-Hunter College HIV/AIDS and Aging Task Force, and a member of both NASW and Hillside Hospital HIV/AIDS committees. She has written a curriculum module for the AIDS Mental Hygiene Project at the School of Education, NYU, and presented on the topic of AIDS and the elderly at several national gerontological conferences.

Mary Ann Malone, C.S.W., is a case manager in the Adult AIDS Unit at Mt. Sinai Hospital in New York. She co-facilitates a support/education group for HIV/AIDS persons over the age of 50 and has given presentations on this topic at professional conferences. She is also an active member of the HIV/AIDS and Aging Task Force.

Marie C. Nazon, M.S., C.S.W., is the Coordinator of the HIV/AIDS and Aging Task Force of New York, Brookdale Center on Aging of Hunter College, and Coordinator of the New York State Best Practices Program in Nursing Homes. She has presented papers on AIDS and aging, family caregiving, and Alzheimer's disease. A return Peace Corps volunteer, she has developed an interest in international aging issues, in particular AIDS and aging in Africa.

Joanne Hanna Puleo, R.N., C, M.S.N., is a Geriatric Clinical Nurse Specialist at Johns Hopkins Bayview Medical Center in Baltimore, Maryland. Formerly of New York, she was a member of the Ulster County HIV/AIDS Consortium and provided home nursing care to persons and families living with HIV/AIDS. She has presented her original work, "HIV/AIDS—Over 50 Facts," at state, national, and international professional nursing conferences.

Karen Solomon, C.S.W., has worked in the field of HIV/AIDS since 1985. At present, she is a consultant for various social service agencies throughout the Northeast. The founding Coordinator/Social Worker for the Spectrum Program at Elder/Family Services, the first federally-funded project to provide targeted mental health and case management services to older adults living with HIV/AIDS, she also provides supervision and training for peer support group facilitators at the People with AIDS Coalition of New York and Lifeforce. She served as co-chair of the HIV/AIDS and Aging Task Force in New York City.

Ron Stall, Ph.D., M.P.H., is an Associate Professor in the Department of Epidemiology and Biostatistics at the University of California, San Francisco. His current research foci include evaluating the effectiveness of AIDS interventions designed for gay men and the behavioral epidemiology of AIDS.

Ann Wyatt, M.S.W., is a Senior Program Associate at the Home Care Associates Training Institute in Bronx, New York, where she is planning an HMO which will serve the severely disabled and chronically ill, including people with AIDS. She was a founder of the Village Nursing Home, Inc. in New York City, and later developed the concept for their AIDS Day Program, which became the first such program in the country.

Chapter 1

Scope of the Challenge

Joanne Hanna Puleo

OVERVIEW OF HIV/AIDS AND AGING

Since AIDS was first recognized in the early 1980s, humankind has been firmly in the grips of a full-blown, ever-evolving pandemic. The enormity and complexity of the actual and potential impact of HIV/AIDS on individuals and their families and on health and social systems worldwide is coming into focus. We are beginning to see that AIDS does not choose who to infect on the basis of sexuality, gender, national origin, or age.

AIDS catapulted into American awareness in June 1981. A group of physicians practicing in the Los Angeles area had filed reports with the Centers for Disease Control (CDC) that described infections associated with immune deficiencies in five homosexual men with no past medical history of immunocompromise (CDC, 1981). Their immune system disorders had somehow been acquired, and despite aggressive treatments the five men died. The story of their deaths, however, would not be an isolated chapter in the history of American health. The story continues to be written to this day and, tragically, may have no end.

The first reports to the public that described this syndrome emphasized a link to homosexual men and their person-to-person transmission through sexual behavior. Then, late in 1981, the syndrome came to be associated with heterosexual injecting drug users, persons with hemophilia, and women, which suggested that transmission was blood-borne as well as sexual.

In 1984, researchers discovered that a retrovirus, which they initially named HTLV III and subsequently renamed HIV-1, was present in the blood and other body fluids of people with HIV/AIDS. An antibody test (see chapter 2) to detect the presence of antibodies to HIV-1 was developed in 1985, and tracking of the incidence and prevalence of HIV seropositivity in populations worldwide began.

The World Health Organization has estimated that 14 million people from the most metropolitan communities to the most remote areas have been infected with HIV. Four million people have developed AIDS (American College of Physicians, 1993). The CDC (1995) reported the number of documented cases of people with AIDS in the United States to be 441,528 through December 1994 and estimated that the number of Americans infected with HIV numbers more than 1 million. Over the next 20 years, the number of HIV-positive (HIV+) Americans is expected to increase to 7 million or more. In the United States, AIDS is the leading cause of death for people aged 25–44 years (CDC, 1994– 1995). As of January 1994, more than 7,500 inmates in 49 separate correctional agencies were confirmed to have AIDS (Criminal Justice Institute, 1994). In New York State prisons, AIDS is the leading cause of death for both men and women of all ages, and it is estimated that as many as 20% of New York's 63,000 inmates are HIV+ (New York State Department of Health, AIDS Institute, 1994). More than 100 people die of AIDS in the United States every day, 1 every 15 minutes (CDC, 1991). AIDS-related health care costs are expected to surpass $50 billion annually by the year 2010. And, unfortunately, this is only the tip of the iceberg.

Although AIDS principally affects young and middle-aged adults, 10% of AIDS cases reported to the CDC have occurred in persons 50 years of age and older (CDC, 1993). In areas where the older adult population is more highly concentrated, the percentage of persons with AIDS (PWAs) who are 50 or older exceeds the national average. Florida's Palm Beach County is one such area in which 15% of PWAs are 50 years or older (Speyer, 1994). The figures describing the incidence and prevalence of AIDS in the older adult population underscores that the virus lives in blood irrespective of the age of the host. Yet public health commentary of the current projected biomedical and socioeconomic consequences of AIDS neglects to address the significance of its impact on the older adult population (Feldman, 1994).

HIV INFECTION

Those infected with HIV and those who will eventually develop AIDS are not found randomly throughout the population. Participating in sexual behaviors with an HIV-infected person, sharing drug use equipment with an HIV-infected person, or receiving a blood transfusion or organ donation from an HIV-infected donor are the behaviors associated with transmission. Mother-to-fetus transmission rates average 25%; however, preliminary results of efforts to decrease this rate through early pharmacologic intervention during pregnancy seem encouraging (Samelson, 1994).

The highest risk behavior associated with HIV transmission for persons over the age of 50 is male–male sex with an infected partner. Nearly 60% of all PWAs in the older adult population were infected by means of this route. Fifteen percent of PWAs who are over 50 were infected by sharing infected drug use equipment. Heterosexual transmission among older adults, nearly unknown before the mid-1980s, rapidly increased by 1990 to 10% of all AIDS cases diagnosed in the over-50 population. This is the largest percentage of heterosexually transmitted cases of AIDS among any age group (Stall & Catania, 1994).

Three percent of all known PWAs became infected as the result of transfusion of infected blood or blood components (CDC, 1993). Older persons are more frequent consumers of health care and are more likely than younger persons to have been infected through blood transfusions. Transmission of HIV-infected blood is associated with 17% of documented PWAs who are 50–64 years of age and with 78% of those age 65 and older (Riley, 1989), and the actual numbers may be much higher. According to the National Academy of Sciences (1986), the potential magnitude of HIV transmission through transfusion cannot be fully predicted owing to the impossibility of testing blood supplies on hand before the availability of the HIV antibody test, which was made available in 1985.

Blood donors who participated in behaviors that indicated that they were at high risk for HIV infection were, before the availability of antibody testing, expected to self-identify through questionnaires or interviews (Clark, 1983). At the present time, interviewing potential donors to screen for those with a history of high-risk behaviors coupled with HIV testing of all donated blood detects an average of 50 HIV-infected donors each year throughout the United States. The New York Blood Center (1995), the largest blood bank in the world, has reported an average of 54 HIV+ donors per year. Despite the strengths of the donor screening and donated blood testing protocols, the system is not perfect. Translated into transmission risk, there remains a 1 in 420,000 chance of becoming infected with HIV through a transfusion (Lackritz, 1995).

EDUCATING PEOPLE ABOUT HIV/AIDS

Educating the public regarding how HIV is transmitted, behavioral risks, and prevention are basic to the effort to reduce infection within all populations. In assessing the effectiveness of broad public education programs, which primarily targeted the hardest hit gay male and young adult populations, the National Health Interview Survey of 1992 (Schoenborn, Marsh, & Hardy, 1994) supplemented its questionnaire with questions related to AIDS knowledge and attitudes. Results of this survey were encouraging in that 93% of Americans reported having at least "a little" knowledge of AIDS. One direct result of the success of the educational strategies used to disseminate information concerning AIDS has been the decline in HIV transmission rates among members of certain gay male communities. Moreover, public discussion of potentially sensitive issues related to transmission and prevention of HIV has become more acceptable. Words such as *condom* and *safe sex* have become commonplace in the American vocabulary. Graphic descriptions and demonstrations of prevention techniques and behaviors have become the norm in many schools, religious institutions, and other community groups.

Unfortunately, older people have not been targeted to receive even the most basic HIV/AIDS information. This is evidenced in the 1992 National Health Interview Survey just discussed, in which 16% of respondents aged 50 and older reported having no knowledge of AIDS. In addition, 77% of these older respondents thought they had no chance of getting the virus. Consequently, they were less likely to seek or give consent for HIV testing. Only 8% of adults over age 50 were tested for HIV in 1992 as compared with 27% of adults aged 18–29 (Schoenborn et al., 1994). The results of the national survey duplicated the results of the survey conducted in 1987 that determined that persons 50 years of age and older generally had a lower level of basic AIDS knowledge than persons in all other age categories (Dawson, 1988). This persistent lack of knowledge of transmission risk coincided with the alarmingly steady increase in the number of AIDS cases among older adults from 1982 to 1991 (National Center for Health Statistics, 1993).

Several possibilities have emerged regarding the health and social policies responsible for neglecting to target older adults for basic HIV/AIDS education despite the significant rise in incidence and prevalence of HIV disease and AIDS within this population. There exists in American society an undercurrent of reluctance, or possibly repugnance, in acknowledging the sexuality and sexual activities of older adults. The practice of stereotyping older adults as asexual grandmas and grandpas is widely accepted. This may be the result of a subconscious Victorian association of sexuality with procreation. Yet, although sexual activity among older adults is likely to be dependent on one's cultural norms, functional abilities, partner availability, and opportunity, sexual expression in the senior years can meet the participants' basic human needs for companionship, physical pleasure, and intimate communication. Despite limited research on the sexual behaviors and activities of the older adult population, rising HIV/AIDS cases within this population demonstrate that older adults are likely to be sexually active and to engage in a variety of sexual activities within a monogamous relationship or with multiple partners (Ryan, Dane, & Tepper 1991). As long as older adults have the ability to make choices in terms of sexual intimacy and other behaviors, they need and deserve inclusion in education campaigns targeting populations at risk for HIV/AIDS infection. Also, because knowledge of one's HIV antibody status is vital to the overall risk reduction effort, older adults need to acknowledge that they are at risk of infection.

The American community is currently experiencing tremendous turmoil and change in the struggle to redefine morality, equality, tradition, family, and the dynamics of relationships over time and lifetimes. Simultaneously, the American population is aging, and acknowledgment of the impact of the older adult on the collective human drama must be made. HIV/AIDS must be recognized as part of older adults' current and future reality. Likewise, the need for immediate action on the part of older adults in matters related to HIV/AIDS necessitates their claiming partial ownership of the expanding tragedy.

Although the variety of HIV/AIDS public educational programs implemented by federal, state, and local agencies have resulted in varying degrees of success in younger populations, they may not prove quite as successful in educating older adults. Learning needs and abilities change as people age. Cognitive efficiency as well as visual and auditory acuity may decline. The need for one-on-one instruction, frequent summarization, and restatement of what is being taught begins to increase as people age. Educating the older adult about HIV/AIDS is further complicated by its negative social stigma and the necessary discussion of sexuality and other topics frequently regarded by older adults as private. Many may "tune out" and fail to recognize that they may be infected. Even though many have recognized the "graying of America," the majority remain relatively ignorant of the diverse composition of the aging society.

In 1995, 44 million persons were over the age of 60, and 14% represented minority ethnic groups. Over the next 30 years, primarily as a result of immigration, the population of older African Americans will grow by 300%, older Hispanics by 395%, and older Whites by 197%. By the year 2030, it is projected that minority elders will total nearly 25% of the older adult population (Harper, 1995). These figures highlight the need not only for educational programs specifically designed for the learning needs of the older person, but for programs that are additionally and progressively culturally sensitive.

Although it is undoubtedly possible to design and implement sensitive multimedia HIV/AIDS educational programs targeted for the older adult, the greatest opportunity for risk assessment and education already exists in the health care setting. Unfortunately, a tendency persists in this setting to neglect taking a sexual history, HIV/AIDS risk assessment, and basic HIV/AIDS education, especially in populations of older adults. Despite the fact that 76% of all Americans visit a physician at least annually, only 15% can recall discussing AIDS during any visit (Gerbert, Maguire, & Coates, 1990). Older adults, as the greatest consumers of health care in this country, average 8.9 physician visits per person per year (National Center for Health Statistics, 1989), yet only 10.8% of persons over the age of 50 have discussed HIV/AIDS with their physicians (Gerbert et al., 1990). As there is presently no cure for AIDS, risk assessment and basic HIV/AIDS education are crucial to the collective effort to contain this virus. Failure to incorporate basic HIV/AIDS education and identification of transmission behaviors into routine and acute health care contacts with older adults deprives them of opportunities for self-care activism in matters related to reduction of risk through behavior modification. In addition, without immediate action, increases in HIV incidence and prevalence in the older population are certain.

It is well documented that older adults have more chronic illnesses and, therefore, more health care and self-care needs than younger adults. Indeed, percentage estimates of older adults affected by chronic illnesses range from 80 to 86% (Fowles, 1989; Office of Technology Assessment, 1985). Yet, 95% of persons 65 years of age or older reside in the community (Carp, 1991), attesting, at least in part, to their pronounced patterns of purposeful health promotion and self-care activities. Although a high level of HIV/AIDS knowledge does not necessarily translate directly into consistent risk-reducing behavior (Baldwin & Baldwin, 1988; Edgar, Freimuth, & Hammond, 1988), research has shown that, overall, older adults are much more likely than younger adults to engage in health promotion activities, particularly when they understand the benefits (Bausell, 1986; Belloc & Breslow, 1972; Levanthal & Prohaska, 1986).

National Institute on Aging (1992) statistics have reported that in 1991 there were, worldwide, nearly half a billion persons over 60 years of age. In the United States, of nearly 250 million people, 12.5% are over age 65 (U.S. Bureau of the Census, 1991). This figure is expected to increase to somewhere between 15% and 16% by the year 2000 (Rempusheski, 1991, p. 6) and to 22% by the year 2030 (Baines & Oglesby, 1991, p. 253). These statistics herald the graying of America and must alert it to all the biomedical, psychosocial, and economic concerns regarding its aging population. The rising incidence of HIV/AIDS in the older adult population is but one of these concerns.

The widespread view that the older population is not at risk for HIV is in stark contrast to the increasing number of older PWAs. Social and health care policy planners as well as primary health care providers must respond to the need for assessment of transmission risk in the older adult population and develop preventative education programs targeting older adults. In a 1994 study of AIDS risk behaviors among late middle-aged and elderly Americans, Stall and

Catania determined that when Americans over 50 are made aware of their risk for HIV/AIDS infection, they can and will modify their behaviors to reduce their risk.

The urgency to target older adult clients for education and assessment of HIV transmission risks and HIV/AIDS knowledge level cannot be overstated. Although this may not be a time for panic, this is certainly a time for action.

REFERENCES

American College of Physicians and Infectious Diseases Society of America. (1993). Human immunodeficiency virus (HIV) infection. *Annals of Internal Medicine, 120,* 310–319.

Baines, E. M., & Oglesby, F. M. (1991). Conceptualization of chronicity in aging. In E. M. Baines (Ed.), *Perspectives on gerontological nursing,* (p. 253). Newbury Park, CA: Sage.

Baldwin, J. D., & Baldwin, J. I. (1988). Factors affecting AIDS related sexual risk-taking behavior among college students. *Journal of Sex Research, 25,* 181–196.

Bausell, R. (1986). Health seeking behavior among the elderly. *The Gerontologist, 26*(5), 556–558.

Belloc, N., & Breslow, I. (1972). Relationship of physical health status and health practices. *Preventative Medicine, 1,* 409–421.

Carp, F. M. (1991). Living environments of older adults. In E. M. Baines (Ed.), *Perspective on gerontological nursing.* Newbury Park, CA: Sage.

Centers for Disease Control. (1981). Pneumocystis pneumonia. *Morbidity and Mortality Weekly Report, 30,* 250–252.

Centers for Disease Control. (1991). Perspective: Changing outlooks. *HIV/AIDS Prevention Newsletter, 2*(3), 1–2.

Centers for Disease Control. (1993). U.S. AIDS cases through September 1993. *HIV/AIDS Surveillance Report, 5*(3).

Centers for Disease Control. (1994–1995). HIV/AIDS advances as leading cause of death for people aged 25–44 in the United States. *CDC HIV/AIDS Prevention, 5*(3), 2.

Centers for Disease Control. (1995). HIV/AIDS cases through December, 1994. *HIV/AIDS Surveillance Report, 6*(2).

Clark, W. A. (1983). Preventing AIDS transmission: Should blood donors be screened? *Journal of the American Medical Association, 249*(5), 567–570.

Criminal Justice Institute. (1994). *The corrections yearbook.* Atlanta, GA: CJI Press.

Dawson, D. A. (1988). AIDS knowledge and attitudes: Provisional data from the National Health Interview Survey. *Advance Data, 163,* 3.

Edgar, T., Freimuth, V., & Hammond, S. (1988). Communicating the risk of AIDS to college students: The problem of motivating change. *Health Education Research, 3,* 59–65.

Feldman, M. (1994). Sex, AIDS, and the elderly. *Archives of Internal Medicine. 154*(1), 19–20.

Fowles, D. (1989). *A profile of older Americans.* Washington, DC: American Association of Retired Persons.

Gerbert, B., Maguire, B. T., & Coates, T. J. (1990). Are patients talking to their physicians about AIDS? *American Journal of Public Health, 80*(4), 467–468.

Harper, M. S. (1995). Caring for the special needs of aging minorities. *Healthcare Trends and Transition, 6*(4), 8–20.

Lackritz, E. (1995, January). *Infectious disease testing for blood transfusions.* Paper presented at the National Institute of Health Consensus Development Conference, Washington, DC.

Levanthal, E., & Prohaska, T. (1986). Age, symptom interpretation, and health behavior. *Journal of the American Geriatrics Society, 34*(3), 185–191.

National Academy of Sciences–Institutes of Medicine. (1986). *Confronting AIDS: Direction for public health, health care, and research.* Washington, DC: National Academy Press.

National Center for Health Statistics. (1989). *Health, United States, 1988.* Hyattsville, MD: Public Health Service.

National Center for Health Statistics, Statistical Resources Branch Division of Vital Statistics. (1993). Deaths from human immunodeficiency virus and detailed subcategories by 10-year age groups, race, and sex: United States 1987–1991. *Work Table, 25,* 1.

National Institute on Aging. (1992). *Global aging.* Bethesda, MD: U.S. Government Printing Office.

New York Blood Center. (1995). [Internal statistics]. Unpublished data reported by D. Kessler, director of the Donor Notification Program.

New York State Department of Health, AIDS Institute. (1994, April). HIV in the prison setting. *Focus on AIDS in New York State,* 1–8.

Office of Technology Assessment. (1985). *Technology and aging in America.* Washington, DC: U.S. Government Printing Office.

Rempusheski, V. (1991). Historical and futuristic perspective on aging and the gerontological nurse. In E. M. Baines (Ed.), *Perspectives on gerontological nursing,* (p. 6). Newbury Park, CA: Sage.

Riley, M. R. (1989). AIDS and older people: The overlooked segment of the population. In M. W. Riley, M. G. Ory, & D. Zablotsky (Eds.), *AIDS in an aging society.* New York: Springer.

Ryan, M. C., Dane, B. O., & Tepper, L. M. (1991). *Attitudes and knowledge of the elderly towards AIDS and safe sex.* Unpublished manuscript.

Samelson, R. (1994). Use of AZT in pregnant women marks breakthrough in epidemic. *Albany Medical Center's AIDS Program Link, 1*(1), 1–2.

Schoenborn, C. A., Marsh, S. L., & Hardy, A. M. (1994). AIDS knowledge and attitudes for 1992. *Advance Data, 243.*

Speyer, R. (1994, March 30). Sexy seniors flirt with AIDS. *The New York Daily News,* p. 6.

Stall, R., & Catania, J. (1994). AIDS risk behaviors among late middle-aged and elderly Americans. *Archives of Internal Medicine, 154,* 57–63.

United States Bureau of the Census. (1991). *Statistical abstract of the U.S.* (111th ed.). Washington, DC: U.S. Government Printing Office.

Chapter 2

Health Care Needs

Kathleen M. Nokes

OVERVIEW OF HIV DISEASE

To work with an older population with HIV/AIDS, it helps to understand the background of the disease itself and how it is transmitted. Retroviruses are a group of viruses that contain ribonucleic acid (RNA), which is changed into deoxyribonucleic acid (DNA) before the virus can become part of the targeted cell in the susceptible person. The change of viral RNA into viral DNA is facilitated through the action of a viral enzyme called reverse transcriptase. HIV disease is caused by infection with a retrovirus (HIV) and host-specific factors that are not yet clear. HIV attaches to host cells that function as a crucial part of the immune system and that have specific receptors. Through this attachment, HIV injects its viral core into the host's immune system cell and subsequently becomes integrated into the host cellular DNA through the action of reverse transcriptase. Once the viral DNA and the host cell DNA become integrated, the person will be infected until death (Hoffman, 1994). The goal of all currently available antiviral medications, such as zidovudine (AZT), is to interfere with the action of viral reverse transcriptase. There are two forms of HIV: HIV-1 and HIV-2. HIV-2 is very rare in the United States, and there are many unanswered questions about how it differs from HIV-1.

HIV-1 enters into an uninfected person's body through body fluids that contain HIV-1. Exchange of sexual and bloody fluids are the most common routes of transmission. The range of time between the point at which HIV-1 becomes integrated as part of the host's immune system cell to the presence of detectable antibodies in the host's blood can range on average from 6 weeks to 6 months. This time period is referred to as the *window period*. During this period, HIV-1 is being trapped by the newly infected person's lymph system (Greene, 1993). It is not known why it takes a relatively long period of time to develop antibodies

9

against HIV-1. Although HIV-infected clients are always infectious, it is believed that they are very contagious during the window period. Most of the newly infected persons will develop a severe, flulike syndrome during this stage of HIV disease.

The Centers for Disease Control and Prevention (CDC) have defined HIV disease a number of times. The latest definition was made effective in January 1993. This description of HIV disease identifies an HIV-asymptomatic stage, an HIV-symptomatic stage (formerly known as AIDS-related complex), and AIDS. An AIDS diagnosis occurs when an HIV-infected client develops one of a potential number of health care problems such as opportunistic infections, unusual cancers, wasting, AIDS dementia, or decrease of a specific type of white blood cell (T4) below 200, or fewer than 14% of the total number of cells. The revised classification system for HIV infection and expanded AIDS surveillance case definition for adolescents and adults is presented in Appendix A. Because it is believed that the amount of HIV-1 virus reflects the extent of the immune system's destruction, clients with AIDS are more infectious than HIV-asymptomatic clients. To summarize, clients are very infectious during the window period when the virus is infecting large numbers of host immune cells and during the end stages of HIV disease (AIDS) when the amount of virus is highest.

The characteristics of infection with human retrovirus are shared with syphilis and Alzheimer's disease, such as long latency periods until major symptoms develop and psychoneurologic signs and symptoms (Schmidt, 1989). Similarities also exist between defects in immunity produced by HIV infection and those manifested by age-related changes (McCormick & Wood, 1992). The most significant aspect of aging-related changes in immunity is decline in cell-mediated immunity, and T cells are the component of the immune system most sensitive to the aging process (Solomon, Benton, Morley, & Temoshok, 1989). The specific type of host immune cell that HIV-1 infects is the T cell.

PRIMARY PREVENTION

Culture needs to be considered in any primary prevention strategy. Culture represents a particular set of values, norms, attitudes, and expectations about the world (Marin, 1991). The HIV epidemic is particularly widespread in communities of gay men and people of color. Organizations such as the Gay Mens' Health Crisis have developed prevention strategies targeted at gay men. Communities of color are very diverse, and a full discussion of the unique needs of each community exceeds the scope of this work. In the Black community, factors generally linked to HIV/AIDS include poverty, homelessness, inadequate housing, fragmented social services, and poor health care, which provide a fertile ground for behaviors that increase HIV transmission (Johnson-Moore & Phillips, 1994). Latinos are one of the fastest growing ethnic groups in the United States (Perez-Stable, Sabogal, Otero-Sabogal, Hiatt, & McPhee, 1992). One of the most important Hispanic cultural characteristics is *familismo*—the emphasis on the family as the primary social unit and source of support. Because of *familismo*, Hispanics may be more highly motivated to talk to other family members about prevention (Marin, 1991). The degree of acculturation is a significant factor (Chachkes & Jennings, 1994) in working with older persons with HIV/AIDS whose country of origin is different from the United States. Cultural values about discussion of sexuality and drug use will affect the design of primary prevention strategies.

To prevent the transmission of HIV-1, infected body fluids should not be exchanged. Many people engage in behaviors that are consistent with possible infection without recognizing that they are placing themselves at risk. Because HIV/AIDS is often unrecognized in the older population, many older people do not believe that HIV/AIDS affects them.

Sexual Transmission

Many older Americans engage in sexual behaviors that place them at risk for HIV infection (Feldman, 1994; Peck 1990). Although older people may be reluctant to talk about a subject that was taboo while they were growing up, it is imperative to ask any client basic questions about his or her sexual behaviors, especially during the period since 1981, in order to determine potential HIV infection. High-risk behavior, such as unprotected sex, by both older men and women includes episodic sexual encounters with paid sex workers of both sexes who know when (Social Security) "check day" is (Joslin, 1994). Condom use is rare among heterosexual middle-aged and older people (Center for Women Policy Studies, 1994).

After menopause, some women experience vaginal changes, including thinning of the vaginal walls, decreased elasticity, fewer secretions, and increased acidity. These women are at higher risk of HIV infection because a dry, thinner vaginal wall is more likely to suffer a microabrasion that can facilitate viral entry (Center for Women Policy Studies, 1994; Wallace, Paauw, & Spach, 1993).

Male–male and bisexual sexual behaviors remain the predominant risk factor for HIV/AIDS until the seventh decade of life (Wallace et al., 1993) but many older homosexual men are very reluctant to "come out" and share information about the gender of their sexual partners (see chapter 6).

In a national telephone survey, it was found that the vast majority of adults were willing to talk about their sex lives when it was demonstrated that the reason for the conversation concerned their own health and the health of people whom they loved (Stall & Catania, 1994). Health care providers need to ask basic questions about sexual practices, using an approach that assumes that the older client will want to share the information. Some examples of questions include, when thinking about the period from 1981 to the present, Were you sexually active? With men, women, or both? Do you use condoms every time, with every partner? Does your sexual partner have any risk behaviors, such as having received a blood transfusion (Weiler, 1990)? Or is he or she a hemophiliac who may have been treated with infected clotting factor?

A sexual assessment should be integrated into the series of other questions about health-related behaviors such as smoking, drinking, exercise, and nutrition. If the client reports any risky behavior, the health care provider should be prepared to teach about barrier protection such as condoms, HIV testing, and, if the client is HIV-positive, partner notification.

Between 10 and 15 years can elapse from time of infection with HIV-1 until death from AIDS, and in some cases even longer periods of health are reported. Some clients in their sixth or seventh decade and older may be particularly reluctant to alter pleasurable behaviors to avoid death from AIDS in the rather distant future. They may feel, especially if they have other chronic, life-threatening illnesses, that the long-term benefits derived from protecting themselves from HIV are not worth the deferred pleasure. Older women may be economically and psychologically dependent on a long-term partner, resulting in a long history of unequal ability to negotiate sexually. They may be resigned to agreeing with the desires of the sexual partner. Again, avoiding a rather distant death from AIDS may be weighed against maintaining a status quo that has evolved over a long period of time.

Injecting Drug Use

Residual blood often remains in the shafts of needles used to inject drugs and can also remain in syringes if blood was aspirated to mix with the drug. Because sharing equipment used to inject drugs often results in injection of not only the drug but also the residual blood, sharing drug-injecting equipment is a particularly high-risk behavior for HIV transmission. It is important to assess if clients have injected any drugs through the skin, especially since 1981. Routes of infection include any piercing of the skin with nonsterile equipment. Stereotypes abound about the characteristics of injecting drug users, and these myths often result in unfounded assumptions. Injecting drug users can hold responsible employment and may have been injecting drugs for 30 or more years. Although these users are probably able to afford sterile equipment, state laws often make access to this equipment very difficult. Examinations of "sterile" syringes bought on the street have found that the packages were resealed. Needle-exchange programs where users can obtain sterile injection equipment have been controversial; they are now growing in popularity in some circles, but are strongly opposed in others. So long as access to sterile syringes remains a significant obstacle, injecting drug use will remain a significant route of HIV-1 transmission.

Because injecting drug use is illegal and can result in imprisonment, an older person may be particularly fearful of disclosure as incarceration is a physically taxing and emotionally stressful experience. The older person may be more willing to admit to unprotected sexual contacts than to honestly discuss a long history of injecting drug use. The provider might encourage the client in this story because the provider may find the active sexuality more acceptable and perhaps even admirable. One of the problems with perpetuating this illusion is that the client is not given information such as the location of needle-exchange programs, which can help to reduce the risk of transmission to others. In addition, other health care problems associated with drug use such as hepatitis B may be missed.

Recipient of Blood Products

Because of life-threatening medical problems, blood transfusions are administered disproportionately to older people. Because there was no blood test for HIV-1 before the spring of 1985, a number of older persons became infected from these transfusions. As the amount of HIV-1 that was transfused was probably relatively large (in comparison to the amount of residual blood that could be found in a syringe), a number of these persons progressed through the stages of HIV disease rapidly and have died from AIDS. Because the blood supply is now being tested for antibodies to both HIV-1 and HIV-2, the risk of infection from blood transfusions is very slight (CDC, 1992). Owing to national blood supply shortages, a client should be reassured that the benefit to be derived from the blood transfusion exceeds the risk of infection because blood is now administered very sparingly.

HIV TESTING

The window period of HIV disease ends with the development of antibodies to HIV. These antibodies are detected in body fluids that contain blood. The two tests for HIV-specific antibodies are the ELISA and the Western blot. In most states in the United States, one blood specimen is tested three times before the results are reported as HIV-1 positive. The first positive ELISA requires a second positive ELISA, which is then confirmed with a more sensitive laboratory test, the Western blot. Older people may be more likely to experience false positive HIV tests because of the presence of other antibodies that might be associated with illnesses common to older people, such as connective tissue disease, chronic renal failure, and hepatitis (Center for Women Policy Studies, 1994). Therefore, it is important to confirm a positive HIV antibody test with a second blood specimen. State laws mandate HIV testing practices and vary greatly from state to state.

Like depression and alcoholism among older adults, HIV/AIDS is often undiagnosed because its symptoms mimic other chronic illnesses associated with aging or because health care providers assume that such symptoms are signs of normal aging. Fatigue, weight loss, and memory and ambulation problems are symptoms of HIV infection or AIDS-related disease that may be misdiagnosed, frequently as Alzheimer's-related dementia (Joslin, 1994). Many health care providers may be reluctant to suggest HIV antibody testing for a variety of reasons that can range from fear of offending the client to assumptions that older people neither are sexual nor use injecting drugs. In light of the growing numbers of older people with AIDS, such failure to assess for risk behaviors and suggest HIV antibody testing could result in malpractice charges as the provider is allowing personal beliefs to interfere with professional judgment.

Although blood testing for HIV antibodies is the most common method, the HIV antibodies can also be found in urine and saliva, and testing for HIV antibodies through analysis of either of these body substances may be available in the near future. Deterrents against making HIV antibody testing too easy include lack of support in the event of a positive reaction and discrimination against the infected person. These factors are being weighed against the reality that only 10% of the population in the United States has consented to blood testing in a setting with a counselor or health care provider.

In addition to antibody testing for HIV-1, direct viral tests, such as polymerase chain reaction (PCR) and viral cultures, are available. These tests can be accessed most easily through participation in a clinical research trial. The direct viral tests are much more expensive than the antibody tests and may never be made available on a widespread basis, but are used in cases where necessary.

SECONDARY PREVENTION

Staging the Client

Because persons with HIV/AIDS could have been infected as many as 15 years earlier, establishing the client's stage of HIV disease becomes important for a number of reasons, including determining when to start treatment, case-finding for HIV-related problems such as opportunistic infections, and estimating prognosis. A surrogate marker, CD4/T4 cell count, has been used to stage clients with HIV disease.

Lymphocytes are white blood cells that consist of a number of subsets including T4 and T8 cells. T4 cells are also known as CD4 cells or as T helper cells. T8 cells are also known as CD8 cells or as T suppressor cells. Normally, a person has twice as many CD4 cells as CD8 cells. Both of these cell types have CD receptors on their membranes, and HIV uses these receptors to inject its viral core into the host cell.

Because of factors yet to be fully explained, the number of CD4 cells decreases and the number of CD8 cells increases the longer a person lives with HIV disease. Depletion of CD4 T cells is associated with increased clinical complications and is a measure of immunodeficiency (CDC, 1994b). The absolute number of CD4 cells is used to make treatment decisions, diagnose when the person has AIDS, and make prognostic decisions (Vedhara, Nott, & Richards, 1995). In some cases, such as an active infectious process, the percentage of CD4 cells is also important to consider. The normal CD4 count may differ between older and younger individuals, and the accuracy of a CD4 count in tracking HIV progression or predicting opportunistic infections in older people may be compromised (Center for Women Policy Studies, 1994). However, although a decrease in lymphocytes is not a normal part of aging, it may occur from malnutrition and a variety of acute and chronic diseases. In those cases, the ratio between T4 and T8 cells is generally normal or increased, and therefore a decrease in the ratio suggests HIV infection even in aged persons (Butler, 1993).

Health Watch is a longitudinal prospective study of healthy aging that uses a computer-based monitoring system for tracking the biochemical, hematological, physiological, and behavioral parameters in men and women (N = 3,000 plus) over their life spans. Normal values of CD4–CD8 cell counts and the ratio between the two values may be different in older clients. In a case study of a relatively healthy 85-year-old person with mild clinical symptoms, T4 cells were 501, T8 cells were 623, and the ratio was .76 in 1984; however, in 1986, T4 cells were 438, T8 cells were 412, and the ratio was 1.06 (Mahler, Schmidt, & Kvitash, 1993). Mahler et al. did not indicate whether the HIV status of this client was ever assessed, so it is assumed that the client was HIV-negative.

Although the waning of cell-mediated immunity seen in aging has not been tied to any particular cell line, T-cell proliferative responses appear to be diminished. A rise in the number of CD8 cells often seen in younger HIV-infected patients is not as vigorous in older patients, which raises concern as there is evidence that CD8 cells are important in suppressing HIV replication and release by CD4 cells (McCormick & Wood, 1992).

The client's stage of HIV disease is also examined through an anergy panel. Cell-mediated immunity is that part of the immune system controlled by T cells. This type of immunity is a delayed reaction; it often takes 48 hours for a significant reaction to be generated. Both persons with HIV disease and older persons develop anergy (loss of responsiveness to skin tests for common antigens such as mumps and tuberculosis; Schmidt, 1989). Approximately one half of uninfected persons over 65 do not respond to the annual trivalent influenza vaccine. Lack of biological response to immunizations is also a concern for persons with HIV disease. Anergy skin testing in older persons with HIV disease may be extremely unreliable because of the decreased functioning of the cellular immune response secondary to both HIV disease and normal aging.

Complications of Treating HIV Disease in the Presence of a Lifetime Pattern of Poor Health Habits

Cigarette smoking has been associated with a more rapid development of *pneumocystis carinii* pneumonia (PCP; Clement & Hollander, 1995). Since the recognition of AIDS, PCP has been the most frequent AIDS-defining diagnosis in the United States and Europe (Hopewell & Masur, 1995). Cigarette smoking is also associated with cervical dysplasia (Becker, Wheeler, McGough, et al., 1994), which greatly increases a woman's risk of developing cervical cancer. Since 1993, the CDC has recognized that cervical cancer, in the presence of an HIV-positive blood test, results in an AIDS diagnosis. An older person who has smoked cigarettes for 40 or 50 years may be particularly reluctant to stop smoking despite the evidence that suggests that smoking accelerates HIV disease.

Older people have established lifelong patterns of eating. As in persons with HIV-related diseases, nutrition plays an important role in immunity within the elderly population. There is a significant correlation between age and immunocompetence with illnesses observed in old age (Zumwalt & Schmidt, 1989). The number of T lymphocytes is related to nutritional status in elderly people (Roebothan & Chandra, 1994).

Factors contributing to nutritional deficiencies include diminished food intake due to pain, fever, or depression; nausea or vomiting due to various forms of drug treatment; dysphagia (difficulty swallowing); dyspnea (difficulty breathing); multiple or chronic physical illnesses; frequent hospitalizations; increased gastrointestinal disorders (such as diarrhea); lower socioeconomic status, which limits food purchases; and dementia (Zumwalt & Schmidt, 1989). Because these factors can occur in both HIV/AIDS and in aging, they can be accentuated in older person with HIV/AIDS.

Complications of Treating HIV Disease in the Presence of Other Chronic Conditions Affecting the Liver and Kidneys

HIV disease affects every part of the body and will complicate the treatment of other physical changes the client may experience. For example, the possible immunodepressive effects of supplemental estrogen and progesterone need to be taken into account if an older woman has HIV disease (Center for Women Policy Studies, 1994).

Gender- and age-related differences in size, weight, and muscle mass should be taken into account in determining treatment dosages (Center for Women Policy Studies, 1994). These issues are discussed fully in the next chapter, which discusses the medical needs of persons with HIV/AIDS.

Disclosure to Preexisting Health Care Providers

Older clients often visit a variety of health care providers such as ophthalmologists or optometrists, podiatrists, and dentists. They may be reluctant to share their HIV status with these health care professionals because of potential embarrassment and fear of rejection. As a consequence, treatment plans will not be suited to reflect the unique needs generated when a person is HIV-positive. A client's response to treatment may therefore be unsatisfactory or a client could actually be harmed by a procedure because added precautions were not taken. To illustrate, a client with HIV disease is at higher risk for bleeding disorders. If a client does not tell the dentist and agrees to an extraction in preparation for dentures, he or she could bleed excessively and require emergency treatment. Even if the client does not have a bleeding episode, healing can be delayed secondary to immune dysfunction, and antibiotics may have been used to prevent infections. These medications are not given routinely, so the provider might not anticipate a problem until a significant infection develops.

Unfortunately, some health care providers do not make clients feel welcome when their HIV status is revealed, so the veil of secrecy persists. The provider's nonverbal behavior can be particularly upsetting if the provider conveys the impression that he or she is shocked or is reluctant to come into contact with the client's blood. As health care providers are required to use barriers such as latex gloves anytime there is a possibility of coming into contact with any client's blood (universal precautions), this should not be an issue. However, a long-term relationship between the health care provider and the client could still be severed.

Manifestations of HIV Disease in Older People

No definitive research has examined manifestations of HIV disease in older as compared with younger persons. The HIV Assessment Tool (HAT) has been described elsewhere (Nokes, Wheeler, & Kendrew, 1994). Data collected to establish the validity and reliability of HAT were used to examine whether any significant differences could be found in severity of HIV-related symptoms and general well-being between older and younger clients with HIV/AIDS. As previously reported, there were essentially no differences in this sample between subjects with HIV disease as opposed to those with AIDS.

An analysis of variance was used to examine differences on each of the 35 items in HAT between two groups: those aged 27–39 years of age ($n = 82$) and those aged 50–68 years of age ($n = 22$). Significant differences were found on 11 items, and in every case, the older clients reported significantly worse symptom severity or decreased general well-being when compared with the younger clients. The older clients reported significantly increased visual problems, difficulty walking, weakness in the extremities, difficulty breathing, sores on the skin, poor appetite, lack of sexual satisfaction, dissatisfaction with life, lack of family and significant other support, and less hopefulness about the future. These findings point to an acute need to examine HIV disease in older clients and to address the unique needs experienced by these persons.

Impact of Prior Lifetime Exposure to Tuberculosis on Combined Effect of Aging Immune System and HIV Disease

Mycobacterium tuberculosis (TB) infection occurs when droplets containing the organism are inhaled by a susceptible person, reach the alveoli of the lungs, and are spread by white blood cells throughout the body. Normally, the person's immune response limits further multiplication and spread, but some of the organisms remain dormant and viable for many years. This condition is referred to as latent TB infection. In general, persons with TB infection have a 10% risk for developing active TB during their lifetime; persons with HIV disease, however, have approximately an 8–10% risk each year for developing active TB (CDC, 1994a).

Persons with latent TB infection usually have positive purified protein derivative (PPD) tuberculin skin test results, but they do not have symptoms of active TB and they are not infectious. HIV-infected persons may have suppressed reaction to PPD skin tests because of anergy. As discussed earlier, uninfected older persons may also be anergic. As a result of the interaction of HIV disease and advanced age, assessing for latent TB infection through PPD skin testing could be unreliable. Determination of whether such persons are likely to be infected with TB must be based on other epidemiologic factors (CDC, 1994a). Residents of long-term care facilities such as nursing homes are considered members of a high-prevalence group.

Latent TB infection is treated with isoniazid (INH), but the risk of INH-associated hepatitis occurs more frequently among persons older than 35 years of age. Therefore, a liver blood test (transaminase) should be done before initiation of INH therapy and monthly during the course of treatment.

Since 1993, pulmonary TB, in the presence of a positive HIV antibody test, has been classified as an AIDS diagnosis. Among elderly HIV-infected patients, most cases of active TB result from reactivation of a latent TB infection that may have occurred years before (Wallace et al., 1993). Any person with HIV/AIDS, especially older persons who have immigrated to the United States, should be questioned directly regarding their prior exposure to TB, perhaps in their country of origin or when they first came to the United States. A diagnosis of active TB should be considered for any person who has a persistent cough (lasting longer than 3 weeks), bloody sputum, night sweats, weight loss, fevers, or loss of appetite. Current recommendations for therapy and dosage schedules for the treatment of drug-susceptible TB should be followed (CDC, 1994a, p. 67). Clients will need assistance in understanding the type and number of pills required and the need to take the medications over a 6- to 9-month period. Interactions between the drugs prescribed to treat TB and other prescription and over-the-counter medications can occur with significant frequency. All of the medications, including methadone, that the client may be taking must be evaluated. A medication schedule should be created because the client can be taking 20–30 pills each day.

TERTIARY PREVENTION

It is widely believed that older persons with HIV disease develop AIDS more rapidly and die more quickly than do younger clients (Ferro & Salit, 1992; Phillips, Lee, Elford, et al., 1991; Ronald, Robertson, & Elton, 1994; Vella, Giuliano, Floridia, et al., 1995; Wallace et al., 1993). Reactivation of dormant infections is more frequent in older people (Center for Women Policy Studies, 1994). One reason for the slower progression rate in younger people may be that, on average, they have been infected with fewer of the opportunistic pathogens that become reactivated during severe immunodeficiency, and so do not tend to develop an AIDS-defining illness as rapidly as do older people (Phillips et al., 1991)

An alternative explanation may be that disease progression appears to be more rapid in elderly persons because of delays in diagnosis (Wallace et al., 1993). Many research studies on women and HIV/AIDS have not even included women over 49 years of age or have not analyzed the data they do have for older women (Center for Women Policy Studies, 1994). Examination of the age of "older" clients in many of the studies reveals a mean age of approximately 40 years of age among the clients who are being characterized as older. In most other contexts, 40 years of age is consistent with the middle years, not the later stages of life. Until prospective research is completed that matches the subjects on a number of variables including socioeconomic status and risk behavior for HIV disease, it seems premature to make any claims about whether there are differences in prognosis based solely on chronological years.

Similarities between the paradigm of geriatric care and the system of care developed for persons with AIDS include use of multidisciplinary teams in care, incorporation of significant others, evaluation of functional and cognitive status, and use of many types of institutional and nonhospital settings for care (McCormick & Wood, 1992). Older people with AIDS often require functional assistance sooner than younger people with AIDS and may require placement in long-term facilities (Schuerman, 1994).

Interfacing with Different Health Care and Social Service Providers

AIDS is the last stage in the continuum that characterizes HIV disease. If the client was evaluated when symptoms of HIV disease first developed, there may have been time to cope with living with HIV disease. The unique characteristics of this last stage result from significant impairment of the immune system, and so the client develops any number of unique health care problems. A client with AIDS can be living with PCP, TB, herpes zoster, or Kaposi's sarcoma. Each one of these conditions requires treatment in addition to the treatment for the underlying HIV disease. Also, the older client may require continued treatment for long-standing health problems such as diabetes or heart disease. As a result, these clients interface with a variety of health and social service providers. The older client with AIDS may access the services provided both to older persons and to people with AIDS and choose among them. To illustrate, an older person with AIDS could choose to receive Meals on Wheels or an AIDS-specific food delivery program, or perhaps both. By qualifying for Medicare, the older person with AIDS may be relieved of the worry of losing health insurance but may find that providers who specialize in geriatrics may not be comfortable with or knowledgeable in treating persons with HIV/AIDS.

Planning for Active Dying—Mobilizing Potential Support Systems

An older person may have lost most of his or her support system, through either AIDS or aging. Many at-home hospice programs require a caregiver who is identified by the client. The older person with AIDS may be forced to enter a residential facility sooner than physically indicated simply because of a lack of social support. There may be concerns about who is left to enact decisions about advance directives such as the health care proxy or living will, funeral arrangements, and burial. Feelings about dying of a stigmatized disease need to be addressed, along with what will be put on the death certificate and communicated in the obituary (Nokes, 1994). Adult children may be particularly embarrassed that their parent is dying of AIDS and request secrecy and concealment. Because death is more expected when older people reach advanced years, there may be fewer casual questions asked about the person's cause of death.

SUMMARY

Although there are many similarities in the health care needs of all persons with HIV disease, there are unique differences when a person is older. There are many unanswered questions about the course of HIV disease in persons who are truly older—not 30 or 40 years of age but 60, 70, 80, or more. The number of cases of AIDS in persons over 50 have been counted for years by the CDC. The age breakdown for the older groups is not easily available, so HIV disease in older persons has not been examined. The similarities between HIV and aging with respect to multiple losses, impairment of immune system functioning, and cognitive changes are striking. One can only wonder why more prospective research has not been completed.

REFERENCES

Becker, T., Wheeler, C., McGough, N., Parmenter, C., Jordan, S., Stidley, C., McPherson, S., & Dorin, M. (1994). Sexually transmitted diseases and other risk factors for cervical dysplasias among southwestern Hispanic and non-Hispanic White women. *Journal of the American Medical Association, 271*(15), 1181–1188.

Butler, R. (1993). AIDS: Older patients aren't immune. *Geriatrics, 48*(3), 9–10.

Center for Women Policy Studies. (1994). *Midlife & older women and HIV/AIDS.* Washington, DC: American Association of Retired Persons.

Centers for Disease Control (1992). Testing for antibodies to HIV-2 in the United States. *Morbidity and Mortality Reports, 41*(RR-12), 1–9.

Centers for Disease Control and Prevention. (1994a). *Guidelines for preventing the transmission of Mycobacterium tuberculosis in health-care facilities.* 43(RR-13), 1–132.

Centers for Disease Control and Prevention. (1994b). *1994 revised guidelines for the performance of CD4+T-cell determinations in persons with HIV infection. 43*(RR-3), 1–21.

Chachkes, E., & Jennings, R. (1994). Latino communities: Coping with death. In B. Dane & C. Levine (Eds.), *AIDS and the new orphans: Coping with death* (pp. 77–99). Westport, CT: Auburn House.

Clement, M., & Hollander, M. (1995). Initial evaluation of and health care maintenance for the HIV-infected adult. In M. Sande & P. Volberding (Eds.), *The medical management of AIDS* (pp. 130–140). Philadelphia: W. B. Saunders.

Feldman, M. (1994). Sex, AIDS, and the elderly. *Archives of Internal Medicine, 154*(1), 19–20.

Ferro, S., & Salit, I. (1992). HIV infection in patients over 55 years of age. *Journal of Acquired Immune Deficiency Syndromes, 5*(4), 348–353.

Greene, W. (1993, September). AIDS and the immune system. *Scientific American, 269,* 99–105.

Hoffman, M. (1994). AIDS: Solving the molecular puzzle. *American Scientist, 82,* 171–177.

Hopewell, P., & Masur, H. (1995). Pneumocystis carinii pneumonia: Current concepts. In M. Sande & P. Volberding (Eds.), *The medical management of AIDS* (pp. 367–401). Philadelphia: W. B. Saunders.

Johnson-Moore, P., & Phillips, L. (1994). Black American communities: Coping with death. In B. Dane & C. Levine (Eds.), *AIDS and the new orphans: Coping with death* (pp. 101–120). Westport, CT: Auburn House.

Joslin, D. (1994). HIV/AIDS and older adults. *CAPCO Capsules, 2*(1), 1–2, 4, 6.

Mahler, E., Schmidt, R., & Kvitash, V. (1993). An artificial intelligence system to predict progression of immune dysfunction in healthy older patients. *Journal of Medical Systems, 17*(3–4), 173–181.

Marin, B. (1991). Hispanic culture: Effects on prevention and care. *Focus: A Guide to AIDS Research and Counseling, 6*(4), 1–2.

McCormick, W., & Wood, R. (1992). Clinical decisions in the care of elderly persons with AIDS. *Journal of the American Geriatrics Society, 40*(9), 917–921.

Nokes, K. (1994). Living with AIDS. In B. Backer, N. Hannon, & J. Gregg (Eds.), *To listen, to comfort, to care: Reflections on death and dying* (pp. 99–117). Albany, NY: Delmar.

Nokes, K., Wheeler, K., & Kendrew, J. (1994). Development of an HIV assessment tool. *Image, Journal of Nursing Scholarship, 26*(2), 133–138.

Peck, R. (1990). An interview with Philip G. Weiler, MD: Why AIDS is becoming a geriatric problem. *AIDS Patient Care, 4*(1), 11.

Perez-Stable, E., Sabogal, F., Otero-Sabogal, R., Hiatt, R., & McPhee, S. (1992). Misconceptions about cancer among Latinos and Anglos. *Journal of the American Medical Association, 268*(22), 3219–3223.

Phillips, A., Lee, C., Elford, J., Webster, A., Janossy, G., Timms, A., Bofill, M., & Kernoff, P. (1991). More rapid progression to AIDS in older HIV-infected people: The role of CD4 T-cell counts. *Journal of Acquired Immune Deficiency Syndromes, 4*(10), 970–975.

Roebothan, B., & Chandra, R. (1994). Relationship between nutritional status and immune function of elderly people. *Age and Aging, 23*(1), 49–53.

Ronald, P., Robertson, J., & Elton, R. (1994). Continued drug use and other cofactors for progression to AIDS among injecting drug users. *AIDS, 8*(3), 339–343.

Schmidt, R. (1989). Biomedical parallels & relationships in research & treatment of HIV- & aging-related diseases. *Generations, 13*(4), 6–14.

Schuerman, D. (1994). Clinical concerns: AIDS in the elderly. *Journal of Gerontological Nursing, 20*(7), 11–17.

Solomon, G., Benton, D., Morley, J., & Temoshok, L. (1989). Psychoimmune connections: Aging, immunity, health, and HIV infection. *Generations, 13*(4), 12–13.

Stall, R., & Catania, J. (1994). AIDS risk behaviors among late middle-aged and elderly Americans. *Archives of Internal Medicine, 154*(1), 57–63.

Vedhara, K., Nott, K., & Richards, S. (1995). Individual variability in the reliability of CD4+ cell counts. *AIDS, 9*(1), 98–99.

Vella, S., Giuliano, M., Floridia, M., Chiesi, A., Tomino, C., Seeber, A., Barcherini, S., Bucciardini, R., & Mariotti, S. (1995). Effect of sex, age and transmission category on the progression to AIDS and survival of zidovudine-treated symptomatic patients. *AIDS, 9*(1), 51–56.

Wallace, J., Paauw, D., & Spach, D. (1993). HIV infection in older patients: When to suspect the unexpected. *Geriatrics, 48*(6), 61–70.

Weiler, P. (1989). AIDS and dementia. *Generations, XIII*(4), 16–18.

Zumwalt, S., & Schmidt, R. (1989). In AIDS & aging: The role of nutrition. *Generations, 13*(4), 77–79.

Chapter 3

Medical Issues

Peter Aupperle

Only modest attention has been paid in the medical literature to the unique aspects of the diagnosis and treatment of human immunodeficiency virus/ acquired immunodeficiency syndrome (HIV/AIDS) in elderly persons. Several articles have hypothesized about the progression of the illness in older adults; however, very few have addressed the critical question of treatment tailored to the physiology of elderly patients. Many published papers have presented case reports of the "unusual" occurrence of AIDS in a geriatric patient, some focusing on the crucial issue of delayed and misdiagnosis of HIV disease. Although several articles have addressed the presentation of AIDS dementia complex in this population, most of this work is based on data from young adults. This chapter summarizes the current extent of medical publications on AIDS and elderly persons and suggests areas of further investigation.

PROGNOSIS OF AGING PERSONS WITH AIDS

As discussed in the previous chapter, the hallmark of HIV disease is the viral infection of CD4+ T cells, which decrease in absolute number during the progression of the disease. These same T4 cells have been shown to have an age-associated decline; hence, it is possible that older age is an independent risk factor for a more rapid deterioration of the immune system. This may result in not only a more rapid progression to the diagnosis of AIDS, but also a decreased survival period (Kendig & Adler, 1990). Several experts have presented data supporting this hypothesis. For example, during one 8-year monitoring of hemophiliac persons infected with HIV, the percentage of progression to AIDS was more than three times greater in adults over the age of 35 in comparison to children and teenagers (Ferro & Salit, 1992). Another study demonstrated that the mean incubation period is 5.5 years for transfusion patients over the age of 59 and 8.2 years for those 59 years and younger (Medley, Anderson, Cox, & Billard, 1987). An additional analysis of people infected by HIV through blood transfusion looked at age at transfusion, sex, and health status at the time of transfusion, and of these variables, only age at transfusion was found to have a statistically significant influence on the latency period from infection with HIV to development of AIDS (Blaxhult, Granath, Lidman, & Giesecke, 1990). It is important to remember that elderly persons are more likely than other age groups to have acquired their infection through transfusion. This may be a second reason for a more rapid progression of HIV/AIDS in older individuals. Some investigators have shown that transfusions are the most virulent mode of transmission, resulting in the shortest survival period for all ages (Ship, Wolff, & Selik, 1991), whereas others have found no difference between the survival of older patients with a history of injecting drug use and those with transfusion-related AIDS (Sutin, Rose, Mulvihill, & Taylor, 1993). Further studies including patients with sexual transmission as a risk factor need to be conducted.

A third cause of shorter survival could be the possibility that AIDS-associated illnesses in elderly persons are more severe, perhaps because of the aging immune system. Inadequate antibody response to immunization against influenza and the greater susceptibility to pneumonia associated with chronic pulmonary and cardiovascular disease are just two of the potential causes of more virulent illness (Kendig & Adler, 1990). Older individuals are also more likely to suffer from malnutrition than are younger adults (Fillit, 1991). For example, it is well-known that mortality due to influenza as well as bacterial meningitis is many times higher in HIV-negative elderly adults in comparison to HIV-negative children. It has also been postulated that an age-associated decline in the rate of T-cell regeneration is to blame for the more rapid progression of infection in older individuals, and this is likely only compounded by the destruction of T4 cells by HIV.

A fourth postulated cause of a shorter survival period in older individuals could be the development of different opportunistic infections than in younger individuals. However, it has been shown that there is no significant difference between those over and under 40 years of age in the percentage of cases with *pneumocystis carinii* pneumonia, Candida esophagitis, or Kaposi's sarcoma as their initial AIDS-defining diagnosis (Sutin et al., 1993). Although this finding could be reexamined with a higher differentiating age, it is noteworthy in that it supports the premise that AIDS in elderly persons is in certain aspects not significantly different than AIDS in younger adults.

A fifth possible cause of premature death in elderly AIDS patients is the underdiagnosis of common medical illnesses because of an inappropriate focus on HIV-related illnesses. For example, case reports exist of older persons with

AIDS who presented with classic signs and symptoms of a myocardial infarction but were misdiagnosed as possible *pneumocystis carinii* pneumonia (McCormick & Wood, 1992). Greater awareness among health care professionals of the need to differentiate the sometimes unique signs of HIV/AIDS in elderly individuals from the signs of other geriatric illnesses will hopefully reduce the likelihood of such errors.

A crucial potential cause of a more rapid progression to death is the known greater toxicity of many antimicrobial drugs in elderly persons. Anecdotal reports have found that older patients are less tolerant of zidovudine (AZT) therapy and have more undesirable effects, perhaps due to the altered rates of absorption, distribution, and clearance seen with most drugs in elderly individuals. This could easily lead to a faster course of the disease. In fact, older AIDS patients have been routinely excluded from clinical trials of new drugs (Adler & Nagel, 1994). This is also reflected in reviews of standard practices of care. One study compared elderly persons with AIDS and young adults with AIDS and found that only 40% of the older cohort compared with two thirds of the younger cohort were receiving zidovudine (AZT; Ferro & Salit, 1992). When retroviral therapy is used in older individuals, the dosage should initially be approximately 50% of the standard adult dose (e.g., 100 mg of AZT every 8 hours, rather than 100 mg of AZT four to five times in 24 hours) to minimize adverse events. However, no studies currently exist examining the relative effectiveness of such dosing (Wallace, Paauw, & Spach, 1993).

HAZARDS OF DELAYED DIAGNOSIS

Finally, a probable cause of decreased survival of older individuals with AIDS is the problem of delayed diagnosis of HIV/AIDS, which clearly can contribute to a poor prognosis. For example, the proportion of AIDS patients who are diagnosed in the same month in which they die increases from about 10% in young adults to about a third of elderly adults (Ship et al., 1991).

AIDS has been called the new great imitator (Sabin, 1987), similar to syphilis decades ago. Numerous case reports exist in the literature of the misdiagnosis of AIDS-related illnesses in elderly individuals and the subsequent delay in appropriate treatments. Several reports have highlighted the frequent treatment of pneumonia in older individuals with standard antibiotics, when they have a presentation consistent with *pneumocystis carinii* pneumonia (Hargreaves, Fuller, & Gazzard, 1988; McMeeking, Schwartz, & Garay, 1989; Rosenzweig & Fillit, 1992).

Often an elderly person presents clinically with a probable pneumonia, and the physician treats it empirically with antibiotics, without obtaining an HIV risk history. At other times a chest X-ray will be done, and despite its consistency with *pneumocystis* pneumonia, the older individual will be assumed to have a severe bacterial pneumonia and still not be treated with the correct medication.

Past diagnostic criteria for AIDS have excluded Kaposi's sarcoma if it occurs in a person over the age of 60, since Kaposi's sarcoma occurred in elderly men before the HIV epidemic. However, case reports have been published in which 75-year-old men have Kaposi's sarcoma associated with HIV infection (Tomasko & Chudwin, 1987). Hence, the current revised diagnostic criteria do not include an age limit, as this has led to misdiagnosis in the past. Of note is the observation that the susceptibility of elderly persons to Kaposi's sarcoma is not associated with an increased incidence of the disease in HIV-infected elderly persons relative to younger HIV-infected cohorts (Boudes, 1991).

In addition, elderly patients have presented with pancytopenia (Boudes, Ballaul, & Sobel, 1989), disseminated tuberculosis (Vadillo, Carbella, & Carratala, 1994), candidiasis (McBride et al., 1992), or chronic gastrointestinal or gynecologic problems as initial manifestations of HIV/AIDS. These illnesses are often assumed to be associated with older age, and appropriate assessments of HIV risk and infection are not pursued. It is essential that all geriatricians be sensitized to the numerous manifestations of HIV/AIDS in elderly individuals.

DIFFERENTIAL DIAGNOSIS FOR DEMENTIA

One of the most challenging and often overlooked diagnoses in HIV-infected elderly persons is AIDS dementia. Given the high percentage of older people with dementia, and the eventual diagnosis of probable Alzheimer's disease in the vast majority of these cases, it is often difficult to diagnose AIDS in an elderly person presenting with purely neurologic signs. In fact, 10% of individuals have neurological symptoms as their initial presentation of AIDS, with about half of these exhibiting purely cognitive dysfunction (Moss & Miles, 1987; Ryan, 1989). The most frequent neurologic disorder is subacute encephalitis, otherwise known as the AIDS dementia complex (ADC). In autopsy series, about 80% of AIDS patients have pathological findings consistent with subacute encephalitis (Fillit, Fruchtman, Sell, & Rosen, 1989).

AIDS dementia complex is a subcortical dementia characterized by a triad of dementia, behavioral difficulties, and motor system dysfunction. Hence, common features include decreased attention and concentration, apathy and social withdrawal, and psychomotor retardation. This differs from early Alzheimer's disease, which is a cortical dementia featuring memory loss, constructional–

spatial difficulty, and associated mild fluent aphasia without neurologic findings (Sabin, 1987). ADC also progresses more rapidly—often over a period of months rather than years. In addition, it is associated with peripheral neuropathies and myelopathies.

Alzheimer's disease patients have no changes in their cerebral spinal fluid; however, ADC patients often have mildly elevated protein levels and a mononuclear pleocytosis. Notable findings on the neurologic examination in ADC are gait ataxia and hyperreflexia, often of the lower extremities (Scharnhorst, 1992). The computerized axial tomography scan of the brain often shows cortical atrophy and ventricular dilitation, and the magnetic resonance imaging scan can show sulcal and ventricular enlargement. The electroencephalogram usually demonstrates nonspecific abnormalities and a generalized posterior slowing (Moss & Miles, 1988).

Finally, ADC is potentially at least partially reversible with the use of antiretroviral drugs that penetrate the central nervous system, whereas Alzheimer's disease is currently irreversible (Wallace et al., 1993). Hence, a case that presents with a precipitous decline of functioning, relatively stronger deficits of attention and concentration, and the presence of psychomotor slowing should be assessed for ADC and dementias other than Alzheimer's (Weiler, Mungas, & Pomerantz, 1988).

SUMMARY

Much more research needs to be done on the medical aspects of HIV/AIDS and elderly persons. These investigations will at a minimum need to include (a) basic science assessments of the virulence and progression of HIV in older individuals with varying risk factors relative to comparable younger cohorts; (b) clinical trials of various antiretroviral drugs in elderly patients to determine appropriate dosing, efficacy, and safety issues; and (c) most important, the education of all health care professionals, particularly those treating primarily older individuals, about the appropriate measures for diagnosing HIV/AIDS in elderly persons (Gordon & Thompson, 1995). The latter seems to be the measure most likely to effect the most rapid and significant change in the survival time of the older patient suffering from this devastating illness.

REFERENCES

Adler, W. H., & Nagel, J. E. (1994). Acquired immunodeficiency syndrome in the elderly. *Drugs and Aging, 4,* 410–416.

Blaxhult, A., Granath, F., Lidman, K., & Giesecke, J. (1990). The influence of age on the latency period to AIDS in people infected by HIV through blood transfusion. *AIDS, 4*, 125–129.

Boudes, P. (1991). HIV infection in the elderly. *Comprehensive Therapy, 17*, 39–42.

Boudes, P., Ballaul, E., & Sobel, A. (1989). Pancytopenia as the presenting manifestation of HIV infection in the elderly. *Journal of the American Geriatrics Society, 37*, 1151–1152.

Ferro, S., & Salit, I. (1992). HIV infection in patients over 55 years of age. *Journal of Acquired Immune Deficiency Syndromes, 5*, 348–355.

Fillit, H. (1991). Reversible acquired immunodeficiency in the elderly: A review. *Age, 14*, 83–89.

Fillit, H., Fruchtman, S., Sell, L., & Rosen, N. (1989). AIDS in the elderly: A case and its implications. *Geriatrics, 44*, 65–70.

Gordon, S. M., & Thompson, S. (1995). The changing epidemiology of human immunodeficiency virus infection in older persons. *Journal of the American Geriatrics Society, 43*, 7–9.

Hargreaves, M. R., Fuller, G. N., & Gazzard, B. G. (1988). Occult AIDS: *Pneumocystis carinii* pneumonia in elderly people. *British Medical Journal, 297*, 721–722.

Kendig, N. E., & Adler, W. H. (1990). The implications of the acquired immune deficiency syndrome for gerontology research and geriatric medicine. *Journal of Gerontology, 45*, M77–81.

McBride, M. O., Maw, R. D., Dinsmore, W. W., Horner, T., Nelson, J. K., & Finegan, O. C. (1992). Acquired immunodeficiency syndrome in the elderly: Two case reports. *Journal of the Royal Society of Medicine, 85*, 240–241.

McCormick, W. C., & Wood, R. W. (1992). Clinical decisions in the care of elderly persons with AIDS. *Journal of the American Geriatrics Society, 40*, 917–921.

McMeeking, A. A., Schwartz, L., & Garay, S. (1989). Don't forget AIDS at any age. *Journal of the American Geriatrics Society, 37*, 1204–1205.

Medley, G. F., Anderson, R. M., Cox, D. R., & Billard, L. (1987). Incubation period of AIDS in patients infected via blood transfusion. *Nature, 328*, 719–721.

Moss, R. J., & Miles, S. H. (1987). AIDS and the geriatrician. *Journal of the American Geriatrics Society, 35*, 460–464.

Moss, R. J., & Miles, S. H. (1988). AIDS dementia. *Clinics in Geriatric Medicine, 4*, 889–895.

Rosenzweig, R., & Fillit, H. (1992). Probable heterosexual transmission of AIDS in an aged woman. *Journal of the American Geriatrics Society, 40*, 1261–1264.

Ryan, F. M. (1989). AIDS as a cause of dementia in the elderly. *Maryland Medical Journal, 38*, 251–254.

Sabin, T. D. (1987). AIDS: The new "great imitator." *Journal of the American Geriatrics Society, 35*, 467–471.

Scharnhorst, S. (1992). AIDS dementia complex in the elderly: Diagnosis and management. *Nurse Practitioner, 17*, 37–43.

Ship, J. A., Wolff, A., & Selik, R. M. (1991). Epidemiology of acquired immune deficiency syndrome in persons aged 50 years or older. *Journal of Acquired Immune Deficiency Syndromes, 4*, 84–88.

Sutin, D. G., Rose, D. N., Mulvihill, M., & Taylor, B. (1993). Survival of elderly patients with transfusion-related acquired immunodeficiency syndrome. *Journal of the American Geriatrics Society, 41,* 214–216.

Tomasko, M. A., & Chudwin, D .S. (1987). Kaposi's sarcoma in an elderly patient. *Annals of Internal Medicine, 106,* 334–335.

Vadillo, M., Carbella, X., & Carratala, J. (1994). AIDS presenting as septic shock caused by mycobacterium tuberculosis. *Scandinavian Journal of Infectious Disease, 26,* 105–106.

Wallace, J. I., Paauw, D. S., & Spach, D. H. (1993). HIV infection in older patients: When to suspect the unexpected. *Geriatrics, 48,* 61–70.

Weiler, P. G., Mungas, D., & Pomerantz, S. (1988). AIDS as a cause of dementia in the elderly. *Journal of the American Geriatrics Society, 36,* 139–141.

Chapter 4

Psychosocial Issues

Karen Solomon

RISK FACTORS AND MISCONCEPTIONS

When dealing with HIV/AIDS and older adults, it is essential that all parties involved address the many preconceived ideas and myths that present obstacles to education, diagnosis, and treatment. The first is that seniors are not at risk for HIV/AIDS because they do not have sex, the second is that persons to whom they are providing services could not possibly have a current or past history of substance abuse, and the third is that persons are most likely heterosexual. It is also important to acknowledge the inherent discomfort of discussing sexual issues with someone who may remind you of a parent or grandparent. Although everyone knows that their parents would have had to have had sexual relations at least once for them to come into this world (as most are too old to have been conceived in a test tube), many have experienced the embarrassment of thinking or hearing about it directly. In addition to the reality of living in a society that does not encourage open discussion of sex, particularly between parents and children, youth-oriented culture encourages the belief that sex is only for the young (Butler & Lewis, 1993). Professionals frequently, and often erroneously, also assume that their clients are heterosexual unless they present overt and obvious characteristics attributed to homosexuality. Many clinicians do not ask the questions that may encourage clients to discuss homosexual behavior and the issues associated with it.

Many clinicians do not acknowledge the existence of alcohol and substance abuse among seniors, either. Sometimes it is simply too difficult to believe that anyone with a history of substance abuse, particularly injecting drug use, can survive into old age. The reality is that due to the tremendous isolation, loneliness, and boredom that can be associated with aging, an increasing number of older people abuse alcohol, prescription drugs, and illegal substances.

Whether at risk from sharing needles or engaging in unsafe sexual behavior while "under the influence," past and present substance abuse presents a very real risk for HIV/AIDS transmission in older adults. It is also rare for health care practitioners to address the issue of transmission through blood transfusions because many of them believe that the risk of receiving an infected transfusion is minimal. In fact, as discussed in chapters 2 and 3, older people have been disproportionately infected with HIV/AIDS through blood transfusions received before 1985 owing to an increased likelihood of prior health problems or surgery.

In addition to failing to recognize that older people are indeed at risk, another factor that prevents timely diagnosis of HIV/AIDS in the older population is the supposition that the symptoms experienced by the aging patient are related to diseases common to elderly persons (McCormick & Wood, 1992). Many older clients have reported that when discussing symptoms with health care providers they are told that what they are experiencing is normal for people their age. Many older people with HIV/AIDS are told that they are overreacting to the normal body changes of aging and that they should just accept them and stop complaining so much. An all-too-familiar story is one in which the elderly person who is suffering from one medical problem after another is compelled to undergo an expensive and exhausting battery of tests, traveling from one specialist to another, only to have the issue of HIV/AIDS ignored until all other possibilities are ruled out. This scenario commonly results in a major delay in diagnosis and treatment. The actual number of older people living with HIV/AIDS is very likely undercounted as a result of misdiagnosis, late-stage diagnosis, and sometimes no diagnosis at all.

The client's own belief system also affects the client–worker interaction. Despite awareness of their own histories, behaviors, and lifestyles, older clients may accept the prevailing assumption that due to their age they are not at risk for HIV/AIDS. Many older clients operate under the assumption that even if they are sexually active, their partner(s) could not possibly be HIV/AIDS-infected because they "look clean," are nice people, or are merely too old. Because many substance abusers (including those with alcoholism) hide their substance use, their partners may be in denial or unaware of high-risk behavior. In addition, many people who are in long-term "monogamous" relationships believe that their partners have been completely faithful, which is not always the case. According to the 1994 survey *Sex in America* by Michael, Gagnon, Laumann, and Kolata, 5% of married partners and 25% of those cohabitating outside of marriage report having had sex with more than one partner within the past 12 months. This population may be involved in one or more of the following behaviors: one or more extramarital/relational affairs, frequenting prostitutes, or participation in anonymous sex or brief sexual liaisons. This includes a number of married men who engage in sex with men outside of their heterosexual relationships, yet do not identify themselves as homosexual or are fearful of being discovered. They are concerned that if they identify themselves as homosexual they will be ostracized by their families and communities and all that they have spent their lives building will be destroyed. This fear of loss and rejection creates an atmosphere of secrecy and lying that affects all aspects of their lives. Many clients who are sexually active outside their long-term relationships do not use condoms with their partners, nor do they inform them of their HIV/AIDS risk or status because they feel they have too much to lose. Instead, they may stop having sex with long-term partners or continue to put partners at risk.

RESPONSES TO DIAGNOSIS

Knowledge of HIV/AIDS status produces a wide range of emotional responses. It is common for people learning of their own or a partner's HIV/AIDS status to react with shock or surprise. This sense of shock is even more pronounced with many older people who, as stated earlier, are under the assumption that they could not possibly be at risk. It is interesting to note that the health care worker providing the HIV/AIDS test result is often as shocked as the client because of these same assumptions. Many of those who have just received an HIV/AIDS diagnosis experience a sense of numbness or lack of reality. They cannot believe that the test result is accurate and are unable to identify or associate themselves with other people living with HIV/AIDS. One older man who had just tested positive for HIV/AIDS responded to the information with the reply "How could this have happened to me? I am not like 'those' people." Many older people with HIV/AIDS and their families have reported that they cannot see or listen to information about HIV/AIDS because it is much too frightening or overwhelming. A common reaction is "Why me?" or "Why now?" Although some speak of having lived a full life and being ready to die, many feel that they are being deprived of time to enjoy their retirement. This is a particularly difficult issue because so many seniors were raised to believe that most of one's adult life is to be spent working hard, saving money, and raising a family. These people spent little or no time participating in leisure or recreational activities while they were actively employed. They believed that retirement was the time of life to enjoy comfort and relaxation and to live out their dreams. Suddenly these seniors who have spent a lifetime looking forward to "the good life" find themselves facing a debilitating, life-threatening illness. Another cruel irony is that many of these older adults have survived other serious illnesses only to be infected by blood containing the HIV/AIDS virus during the treatment of these ailments. This can result in a tremendous sense of mistrust and anger toward the health care system.

Stigmas and Secrecy

Many seniors affected by HIV/AIDS are afraid to seek assistance and support because of both the stigma associated with the disease itself and the risk behaviors associated with transmission. Although all people living with HIV/AIDS face stigma and rejection, older people were raised during a time when many of the behaviors associated with HIV/AIDS were highly stigmatized and considered ugly family secrets.

Before the 1960s, issues such as sex, sexuality, alcohol and substance use, expression of feelings, and basically any deviation from the norm were met with distrust and were not openly discussed. The prevailing attitude was that one "kept one's dirty laundry to oneself" and that if these issues were to be discussed at all they were to be kept within the family. Being stoic, tight-lipped, and independent when facing problems were valued, and only "crazy people" sought therapy. Sex was not something one talked about, and homosexuality was an issue still in the closet, along with many of the people who lived that lifestyle. Only the local bum on the corner was an alcoholic or addict; Uncle Joe "just liked his beer." Doctors and other professionals were perceived as having all the answers, and one did not question authority.

It must be acknowledged that the 1960s brought a major revolution in communication within society. Support, encounter, and assertiveness training groups encouraged people to share private issues and feelings with people outside of the family. An increase in substance use led to the development of many drug treatment programs and publicized the already existing 12-step programs. A widespread acknowledgment of the prevalence of alcohol and substance abuse in this culture began to emerge. The Stonewall riots in the summer of 1969 initiated the increased visibility of homosexual men and homophobia. In the decades following, these and other issues have been addressed in movies, magazines, talk shows, and other mass media, resulting in a normalization of the topic of homosexuality, if not outright acceptance by the larger society. Many of those who came of age during and after the 1960s became part of a culture that valued discussion and sharing of feelings. Therapy and group participation were perceived as routes to support, personal growth, and change, and differences were acknowledged, in varying degrees, as a reality in this society.

A large number of older adults did not participate in many of these changes.

For them, discussing feelings or asking for help outside of the family continues to signify weakness. They feel the stigma of HIV/AIDS even more intensely than most because many of their contemporaries continue to judge the behaviors associated with HIV/AIDS as being morally wrong. In addition, a substantial number of these clients are involved in religions that also judge these behaviors as morally wrong and consequently reject people living with HIV/AIDS. Those involved in organized religion frequently receive the message that HIV/AIDS is a punishment from God and that they are paying for behaviors deemed immoral. For those who turn to religious leaders and communities for support or assistance, the response has sometimes been less than positive. Although some HIV/AIDS-affected individuals have received tremendous support and love from fellow believers, others have met with rejection or outright condemnation. These factors contribute to an environment of isolation, secrecy, and lies. Some people refuse to tell their families and friends until it becomes absolutely necessary, and others never tell. In one case, a man who lived through various forms of cancer had received an HIV/AIDS-infected blood transfusion. His family doctor, who had been treating this man for many years, informed the man's wife. She and the doctor decided that the man could not face the shame and stigma of an HIV/AIDS diagnosis. In the words of the wife, "it would kill him." He died never knowing his HIV/AIDS status. In another case, a woman who had received an infected transfusion during cancer treatment responded on learning of her HIV/AIDS diagnosis, "What will people think of me? What will they think that I did? They won't want to put their laundry in the same machines that I use." She had been very vocal and outspoken about living with cancer, but insisted to her family that they lie and tell everyone that she had cancer, not HIV/AIDS.

Clearly, the secrecy that many experience regarding an HIV/AIDS diagnosis is very complicated and confusing for all involved. It is difficult to remember who knows the truth and what each person has been told. Secrets also make it difficult to reach out for support and services. There is concern about being identified merely by entering into the offices of a program that provides HIV/AIDS services. What will the neighbors say if they see a nurse or social worker walking into the home? Many older clients have major concerns about confidentiality and accessibility of records. It is vital that workers take the time to discuss these issues as well as the safeguards that are available and can be put in place. Sometimes workers feel frustrated or impatient about all of this concern for privacy and secrecy. It is important to remember that people have, in fact, lost jobs, homes, and family and have been subjected to social isolation and rejection because of their HIV/AIDS status. Therefore, it is not helpful or fair for workers to minimize these concerns.

Guilt and Shame

Because of the risk behaviors associated with exposure to HIV/AIDS, many clients experience tremendous guilt and shame following their diagnosis. There is major concern about being judged for activities in which they may or may not have been involved. One still hears talk about innocent victims. Children and those who were infected through blood transfusions are judged as the innocent, whereas others are perceived as deserving their predicaments. This blaming that takes place leads many older adults infected with HIV/AIDS to remain isolated from the general aging population as well as the HIV/AIDS community. Many older adults who have sought assistance from HIV/AIDS organizations have reported that they feel different from most of the people who use the services. In addition to the prejudice and judgment with which older persons perceive the other clients, they feel that these people are too young and their issues too different to understand. Other people deal with HIV/AIDS with tremendous denial. In an "out of sight, out of mind" approach, these older adults believe that if they do not think about or allow themselves to experience their feelings, they will not be affected by HIV/AIDS. For others, the fear that is associated with a diagnosis of HIV/AIDS gets expressed as anxiety about the future and how the illness will affect it. For many, their worst fears of physical and mental debilitation, dependence, depletion of financial resources, suffering, and a prolonged, painful death become a very real and frightening possibility.

GETTING HELP

Emotional

Given the reluctance that many older adults have about discussing feelings, asking for help, and especially becoming involved with mental health professionals, it may be helpful for workers to approach potential clients by offering assistance in obtaining concrete services. Some people in need of support may feel insulted by the suggestion of therapy and not understand what takes place in support groups. Many of these individuals need to believe that they are perfectly capable of handling the situation on their own and are uncomfortable with feeling vulnerable or "weak." Provision of concrete services can serve to create a nonthreatening access point for workers and allow clients to begin to establish a trusting relationship that can expand over the course of time. One client described this process to another potential client in this way:

Oh, you don't have to worry about Ms. X, she's there to help you with your problems. If you have a problem with your electric bill, she can help you know what to do. Also, if you have a problem, you can talk to her about anything. It's good to talk about your problems, you feel better.

Financial

Older adults living with HIV/AIDS do in fact face a myriad of financial factors and complications that differ from those faced by the younger population. Many seniors are retired and living on fixed incomes, including social security, pensions, and savings from retirement accounts. The astronomical costs of medical care and treatment can wipe out or diminish savings, particularly for those with little or no insurance. McKinlay, Skinner, Riley, and Zablotsky (1989) offered that an AIDS diagnosis often means economic dependence. Many of these older clients have major fears and concerns about spending the money they have saved for years to pay for medication and home care. Particularly for those who lived through the depression, there is a strong belief that money in the bank represents security and that the loss of this money will result in destitution and homelessness. Others feel that they have worked and saved their entire lives in order to be comfortable and to leave a legacy for their children and grand-children. These seniors experience frustration and anger at the prospect of wiping out their savings to pay for medical costs. Medicare, which is available to all U.S. citizens over the age of 65, provides limited medical and prescription coverage. This leaves a balance that patients must cover themselves. With the multiple medical problems associated with HIV/AIDS, the patient's share can total thousands of dollars over the course of a year. In addition, savings and benefits received by seniors often render them ineligible for Medicaid coverage. Most private insurance covers only part of medical and prescription costs. For those who are eligible, veterans' hospitals and centers offer free or low-cost treatment as well as prescription coverage. To effectively assist older adults in negotiating benefit and entitlement systems, workers must be well informed and up to date on the various regulations and restrictions that are involved.

PERSONAL REACTIONS

Although the older population appears to be knowledgeable about HIV/AIDS transmission, a recurring theme for many older HIV/AIDS-affected clients is fear of transmission through casual contact. This is a particular concern as it relates to grandchildren. One client refused to hug or allow his grandchildren to have any physical contact with him. He reported that he could not stand the thought of his grandchildren getting "this terrible disease" because of him. Frequently, an initial reaction of older people infected with HIV/AIDS and their caregivers is to limit contact with family members or to use disposable dishes, cups, and utensils to protect loved ones from the virus.

Many people are able to move through this stage with education and assistance in coming to terms with their feelings. In addition to the distancing that results from a fear of contagion, a strong similarity between the aging process and HIV/AIDS is that many people are uncomfortable in facing the physical realities caused by these conditions, which may include deterioration, pain, disability, helplessness, and sometimes disfigurement. Some people who are not able to deal with these feelings maintain an emotional or physical distance from loved ones affected by HIV/AIDS as the person with HIV/AIDS becomes increasingly symptomatic and debilitated. At this point, loved ones may begin avoiding the person with HIV/AIDS because they are unable or unwilling to watch the process of deterioration or face the pain of losing him or her. This is similar to reactions to the aging process, when family members who find it difficult to watch the changes in physical and mental status avoid contact with the older person. Offering family therapy, support, and assistance is essential for all families facing HIV/AIDS.

Another issue is the reaction of loved ones to the risk behavior itself or the feelings associated with being infected by someone you love. One 70-year-old man tested HIV-positive and identified his risk behavior as repeated sex with high-risk prostitutes. His wife was immediately tested and also tested positive. The wife was so hurt and angry about her husband's high-risk behavior as well as his lack of protection of her from HIV/AIDS that she forced him to leave their home and insisted that he not have contact with his children or grandchildren. At the time of this writing, this man lives completely isolated and alone in a rooming house in another part of the state. Each time he has attempted to contact his daughter to get a picture of his grandchildren he has been rejected. When he asked to see his grandchildren from across a shopping mall without their knowledge, his daughter refused him. He has had no further contact with his family.

In addition to the sexual issues that are common in long-term relationships, couples with one or more partners who are living with HIV/AIDS face increased difficulties. Partners dealing with HIV/AIDS must deal with the fear that sexual activity may result in transmission of HIV/AIDS to a loved one. Even when partners are well informed about safer sex there is often tremendous fear of transmission. This can result in a complete lack of sexual activity that can leave the partner with HIV/AIDS feeling like a pariah, rejected, unlovable, and frustrated. In addition to the fears associated with sex in an HIV/AIDS-affected relationship, sexual desire is also directly affected by HIV/AIDS. Depression, side effects of medication, fatigue, and other symptoms can reduce or eliminate sexual desire and functioning. Workers must be willing to raise issues of sex and sexuality with older clients living with HIV/AIDS in order to normalize and address issues such as continued high-risk behavior, intimacy, homosexual lifestyle or behavior, relationship problems, sexual desire, and dysfunction.

LOSS

Aging can also bring many other changes in lifestyle. This may include loss of status, limited income, and a decrease in the daily activity level following forced or voluntary retirement. For some elders, the process of adult children maturing and living their own lives, moving out of the home, or living far away creates a very real sense of separation and loss. The once head of household must now adapt to a loss of status and the feeling of no longer being important and needed by loved ones. Aging also brings with it the death of loved ones. Many older adults are already grieving the loss of parents, spouses, siblings, friends, and other supports, which adds to the feelings of loneliness, abandonment, and isolation. Aging, as well as HIV/AIDS, brings on a variety of body changes that can be experienced as loss. These include loss of overall health, increasing aches and pains, and decreasing energy. Changes in physical appearance, already a painful issue, are further compounded by the Western ideal of beauty, which is identified with youth, physical vitality, and glowing health. For many, the aging process has resulted in limited mobility and an increased amount of time spent isolated in the home. This may be due to arthritis, poor health, fatigue, limited social networks, retirement, fear of danger or violence in the streets, and other factors. Becoming homebound due to increasingly debilitating symptoms and fatigue can become the unfortunate reality, particularly for older adults living with HIV/AIDS.

The actual or potential process of physical and mental deterioration raises many issues of dependence for older adults affected by HIV/AIDS. For some, these issues include shame and embarrassment about not being strong, independent, or in control. For others, this loss of independence stimulates concerns about being a burden on loved ones or fearing that nobody will be able or willing to assist them if necessary. It must also be noted that for many seniors HIV/AIDS is a compounding isolating factor that creates an atmosphere in which television, radio, newspapers, and magazines are the main or only source of contact and communication with the outside world.

PROGRAMS AND OUTREACH

Given the reality of impaired mobility for many of these older clients in need, it is essential that programs attempting to reach this population provide home visiting services as well as case management to assist clients and their families in obtaining a range of home care services. As the need for assistance and services in the home increases, there is the issue of invasion of privacy, particularly by strangers. Older adults who have spent much of their lifetime being independent and self-sufficient become set in their ways and find it difficult to adjust to the presence of home attendants, social workers, nurses, and others on a regular basis. Because of the extensive number of hours that home attendants and home health aides spend with the clients, these relationships can easily become a source of tension and conflict. It is important for the health care worker to understand the dynamics of the situation, including feelings of loss of privacy, independence, and control. Even family members who are present in the home on a regular basis report conflict because this "outsider" is taking control of the care of their loved one. They often believe that the care given by the home attendant or home health aide is not as good as the care that they could provide if they were able to.

Many older adults with HIV/AIDS experience prolonged bouts of depression and persistent anxiety. They are forced to face many anxiety-producing questions, including "What will I ultimately be capable of?" "Will I be dependent on someone to take care of me?" "Will I have the finances I need to survive?" "Will I be a burden on my loved ones?" and "Will I have to suffer?" Clearly, these are difficult and painful issues. A common reaction to dealing with the fear of the future is suicidal ideation, planning, or both. Older adults living with HIV/AIDS express fear of deteriorating into a vegetative state. When asked, many are able to identify the point at which they would no longer want to go on and describe in detail how they would kill themselves. This author has found that when clients are allowed to discuss their concerns openly, feelings of control increase. This feeling is particularly important when dealing with HIV/AIDS issues where control over one's body is frequently not possible. When allowed the control over the prospect of limiting their suffering, these clients often express a sense of relief and are able to focus on living in the moment. It is almost as if they feel that they are now choosing to live instead of helplessly existing in a process of death and deterioration. In reality, most people do not decide to kill themselves when they reach this predetermined point; many struggle to take every last breath that they are capable of.

It is the primary task of health care workers to openly and honestly address issues regarding death and dying and the role of the health care worker in the process. Although many come to this work to help people improve the quality of their lives, it may not always be simple to evaluate one's efforts. HIV/AIDS, as well as advanced aging, can make it difficult to notice the quality of life present in the midst of physical or mental deterioration, suffering, and pain. It is essential to come to terms with one's own feelings of helplessness and accept the fact that sometimes all one can do is to continue to be present for that person and, more often than not, to be one of the few people willing to have some kind of physical contact.

Communication

It is also important for workers to be aware of their own expectations about older clients dealing with HIV/AIDS. For example, the language of affect and feelings is one that is not necessarily familiar to some of this population. Frequent responses to the inquiry "How are you feeling?" include "How do you think I am feeling?" "How would you feel if you were me?" "Fine," "Better," "O.K.," or "Lousy." Sometimes the communication is difficult because individuals are not aware of or connected to their feelings; other times they may feel uncomfortable sharing painful or difficult feelings with someone who is perceived as an outsider or stranger. It is important to create an open, relaxed, and accepting atmosphere from the onset. This involves allowing the client to discuss any issue with which he or she is comfortable, including current events, game shows, the weather, and so forth. Many older clients are so uncomfortable communicating with a health care worker that they may leave the radio or television on during the entire home visit. As long as the sound is lowered and does not serve as a total distraction, leaving the TV or radio on may help the client feel more in control of the environment during the session. Another helpful technique is to reflect on feelings that are being expressed directly or indirectly. At some point in the relationship, the older client who is experiencing the progression of illness associated with HIV/AIDS may lash out in anger or frustration at the worker who is perceived as "useless" if the client feels that needs are not being met. This is an excellent time to reflect on feelings of anger, frustration, and helplessness regarding the situation and the disease. In one situation, an older man with HIV/AIDS who had been bedridden for more than a year was being very hostile to the worker, telling her she was stupid when she responded to a question he had asked. She asked him, "Are you mad at me?" He hesitated and said, "No. Why do you ask?" She replied, "Because you sound angry and just called me stupid." He said, "I am angry. Angry at what is happening to me, angry that I am getting worse, and angry that nobody can help me." Before this discussion, this man would only talk about current events and the weather. If such a clear opportunity does not arise, an intervention that suggests or normalizes feelings may be in order. This can include approaches such as "If I were in your shoes I would feel . . ." or "A lot of people I know are experiencing things similar to what you're going through and they tell me they feel. . . ." It is also may be necessary to ask open-ended as well as leading questions in order to elicit discussion. One of the most basic aspects in the development of trust between the older client with HIV/AIDS and the worker involves consistency. In addition, the worker must show up, be emotionally present and caring, and provide assistance in obtaining support, services, and benefits.

Professional Limitations

It is also necessary for health care workers to be aware of their own limitations and that one of their primary responsibilities is to serve as witnesses to another being's living, suffering, and dying. This can be extremely painful, but it is very important. Frequently, it is the health care worker's role to help the person die with dignity and a sense of closure. This entails filling out living wills, do-not-resuscitate orders, powers of attorney, health care proxies, wills, and other advance directives (see chapter 8). It may involve contacting and speaking with loved ones and friends. It also means being receptive to the client's desire to discontinue medications, eliminate tube feeding, and not receive further treatment. At this point, it is important to explore hospice care with the client and relatives.

Support Systems

This process of letting go and dying is greatly affected by the individual's spiritual beliefs and support system. In this author's experience, many of those who have a strong belief in some form of a "higher power" or God are able to face the prospect of suffering, pain, and death with a sense of faith in a bigger picture. In addition, some are able to find comfort and hope in the belief of an afterlife or reincarnation. A strong support system is also essential to the grieving process. Family, lovers, friends, and helping professionals can help the older person with HIV/AIDS to feel that he or she is not alone and may feel free to discuss often frightening and painful feelings. This support can serve as a powerful component of an accepting and expressive grieving process.

COPING SKILLS

Older people with HIV/AIDS do develop and use a wide range of coping skills in living with this disease. As stated earlier, religious beliefs and acceptance by the community are helpful in this area. Many people use coping skills that they have developed from knowledge and experience accumulated over a lifetime of trials and tribulations. For some, these decades of surviving, watching, and participating in history provide a sense of perspective and acceptance that younger individuals do not have access to. For other older adults affected by HIV/AIDS, this crisis provides an opportunity to learn new skills and methods of addressing issues. This can include reaching out and asking for support, an increasing honesty with oneself and others, acquiring new communication skills, and appreciating what one has in one's life as opposed to what is missing. Clearly, HIV/AIDS can also be a powerful force that can divide or bring family members together. Some families have been destroyed by shame, anger, stigma, and fear in relation to the member living with HIV/AIDS, and others have overcome tremendous interpersonal and logistical obstacles to be present for their loved one with HIV/AIDS. There is also a group of these HIV/AIDS-affected older adults who become very active in their own health care process. These individuals acquire as much information as possible about HIV/AIDS treatments, infections, and services and become self-advocates with health and social service professionals. Others become outspoken activists and leaders, increasing awareness about older adults with HIV/AIDS and advocating for increased services.

SUMMARY

Health care providers must begin by challenging ageist assumptions and misinformation that impede efforts to educate, treat, and provide services to older people living with HIV/AIDS. It is up to these providers to be aware of the particular needs and concerns of this special population. To effectively assist these clients in facing difficult and painful issues associated with HIV/AIDS, as well as aging, it is essential that health care workers take the time to address their own responses and levels of comfort when addressing these same issues. Health care workers must use their role as part of a support team that includes friends, family, loved ones, and other professionals to help reduce feelings of isolation. It is possible that during a time of great loss, stress, and pain, health care workers can assist clients to explore new aspects of themselves and help them to maintain a sense of self-respect and dignity.

REFERENCES

Butler, R., & Lewis, M. I. (1993). *Love and sex after 60.* New York: Ballantine.

McCormick, W. C., & Wood, R. W. (1992). Clinical decisions in the care of elderly persons with AIDS. *Journal of the American Geriatrics Society, 40,* 917–921.

McKinlay, J. B., Skinner, K., Riley, J. W., & Zablotsky, D. (1989). On the relevance of social science concepts and perspectives. In J. B. McKinlay, K. Skinner, J. W. Riley, & D. Zablotsky (Eds.), *AIDS in an aging society* (pp. 127–143). New York: Springer.

Michael, R. T., Gagnon, J. H., Laumann, E. O., & Kolata, G. (1994). *Sex in America: A definitive survey,* (pp. 100–103). Boston: Little, Brown and Company.

Chapter 5

Creating a Support Group

Barbara Kornhaber
Mary Ann Malone

The impact felt by older adults at the hands of HIV infection is profound. The impact of this infection on the over-50 population is extreme for many reasons. Not only must this population cope with the "normal" physiological aspects of the aging process such as reduced ability to ward off infections, the general decreased functioning of the body, the decreased ability to remember, and the physical toll that aging exacts on the body, but they must also cope with the stigma of HIV infection (Layzell & McCarthy, 1992). This is compounded by complexities produced by delayed identification of HIV disease. HIV disease may progress more rapidly in elderly persons, but it is also possible that the observed shorter survival time may result from a delay in diagnosis (Wallace, Paauw, & Spach, 1993).

The difficulty in accepting HIV disease in this age group by the members of the group itself is a problem that is mirrored in the professional and nonprofessional community as well. As a result of the disbelief, denial, or reluctance to recognize the presence of HIV in the over-50 age group, there are patients for whom earlier diagnosis would perhaps have avoided many problems. These problems include premature deterioration, acute discomfort, much unhappiness, and possibly one or more hospitalizations. Help and assistance can be provided through early diagnosis. By shortening the time it takes to diagnose HIV infection, the course of the infection can be influenced. Prognosis could also be improved by providing treatment suitable for elderly persons (Dupon, Bismuth, Parneix, Morlat, & Malou, 1991). Not only could early diagnosis lead to earlier treatment, but supports for handling the psychological impact of the illness could also be put in place. As mentioned previously, older persons experience many physiological losses, and receiving an HIV diagnosis can only compound the existing sense of loss. The overriding goal of any intervention following a loss is to assist an older individual to achieve the highest quality of life possible (Conway, 1988).

Exploring the issue of HIV and AIDS and aging generated a number of questions:

- Can the HIV-infected population over the age of 50 benefit from the use of a support group?
- Were these older HIV-infected people struggling with loneliness, sadness, guilt, and isolation?
- Did they have questions about the progression of their illness or about the medications they were taking?
- Were they aware of the benefits to which they were entitled?
- Did they see themselves as victims of an uncontrollable disease?

The authors decided that they would create services to assist them in obtaining mutual support for their psychological needs and to provide education and answers for questions they had related to their illness. They would also be available to assist with referrals for concrete service needs. Gallo (1982), in his study on the value of support networks for elderly persons, showed a positive relationship between strong support networks and the status of elderly persons' health. Harel's (1988) article indicated that support networks could assist in the reduction of disease symptoms and that older people who had more informational support and who provided support to others had fewer symptoms of depression.

There is very little written about support groups for older adults with HIV/AIDS, which indicates an insufficient appreciation of their needs. Most of the literature the authors reviewed dealt with the older population in general, support groups for that population, and support groups for non-age-specific persons with HIV/AIDS. In this chapter, the experience of starting and facilitating a support–education group for persons over the age of 50 who have HIV/AIDS is explored and evaluated. The authors have drawn on what they have read to assist in their efforts to provide an atmosphere of mutual support for these older people.

At present, there is only one other organization in the New York City area that offers support groups for older HIV-infected persons. Senior Action in a Gay Environment (SAGE) conducts three support groups for older homosexual men. The scope of the SAGE groups is mandated and therefore limited by the population of its members and dictated by their common experiences. (This program is presented in detail in chapter 6.) The intent of the authors' project was to see if the success that is being experienced by the SAGE groups could be duplicated with a mixed heterosexual–homosexual, male–female population.

A support and education group can provide help in many areas. A support group is a proven modality to help the individual to identify and explore areas of concern in the environment primarily composed of his or her peers. Combining support with education enhances the ability to deal with issues that either may unexpectedly arise or can be predicted.

CONCEPTUAL FRAMEWORK

The model used in the educational piece of the project was based on the work of Betz, Wilbur, and Roberts-Wilbur (1981). A discussion-format group type is designed to facilitate the working out of feelings in the guise of an educational growth group (Cerio, 1979). The educational growth group allows for the provision of information to group members and opportunities for clarifying values, for experiential learning, and for future planning. Many of the issues that surface with the older population deal not only with physiological changes but also with the numerous psychological manifestations and stresses resulting from loss.

Green (1990) suggested that a number of characteristics and circumstances are shared by many older people: (a) loss of status, resulting in an increased uncertainty about personal worth; (b) insecurity associated with feelings of an inability to meet the demands of life; (c) apprehension about health; (d) having a very difficult time adjusting from a work routine to a routine of retirement; (e) difficulty in finding an avenue of service that will provide personal gratification; (f) difficulty in handling stress created by social change; and (g) limited incentive for social participation.

The problems shared by almost all elderly persons are complicated and compounded by HIV disease. Gathering together a group of individuals who share the same difficulties or the need to deal with similar changes in their lives brings out the "lifeboat" mentality in them (Alcoholics Anonymous, 1939). The commonality that is inherent in their shared experiences creates a bonding that may surpass all of the participants' previous experiences.

FACILITATORS' APPROACH

There are several ways to approach working with groups of older persons. One is a time-limited, task-oriented approach with specific goals. Leadership for this type of group is more directive. Another approach focuses more on the group process, with less directive leadership and a more open-ended time frame. Both approaches aim to achieve the same goal: mutual support for group members. Most of the literature has indicated that the open discussion type of format is more effective in helping elderly persons. Toseland, Sherman, and Bliven (1981), in their study with four experimental groups using these two approaches, found that members of the highly structured group did not like the directive approach mainly because it reminded them of school. They preferred a less directive approach with the group leaders acting more to facilitate process. Because the purpose of the group formed by the authors concentrated on support and education, the authors felt the process-oriented approach was a more appropriate method to facilitate a group of older persons with AIDS-related concerns.

GETTING ORGANIZED

Once the questions were identified, the literature researched, and a need established, the authors decided to determine if there was a population large enough to warrant pursuing this project. Both authors were employed by a 1,200-bed teaching hospital and medical center that serves the Upper East Side and East Harlem in New York City. This geographical area has a predominantly African American (including Haitians), Hispanic (including South Americans), and White (including recent immigrants) population. The outpatient Infectious Disease Clinic serves people with many infectious diseases, but primarily those who have been diagnosed with HIV infection. The New York State Department of Health has identified the tertiary care facility as a designated AIDS center.

To identify if there was an adequate population for a group, the authors requested a computer search of the 1,003 patients with HIV disease who were being treated at the Infectious Disease Clinic. One hundred four (10.3%) were identified as being over the age of 50, a percentage that reflects the national average of people over 50 years of age who are HIV-positive. Of this group ($N = 104$), 38 (36.5%) were appropriate for inclusion in the support–education group, of which 24 (66%) were men. Factors that determined appropriateness for inclusion in the group were physical mobility, mental status, psychiatric history, ability to communicate in English, and availability.

Physical mobility was an issue as transportation could not be provided. Each potential member of the group needed to be able to attend each meeting and return home independently. The public transportation system is quite extensive in the area surrounding the hospital. Mental state was important as each member needed to be able to participate actively in group discussions. Because this was not to be a psychopathologically oriented group, any extensive psychiatric history or current psychiatric diagnosis or problems eliminated a potential group member. The ability to communicate was important in order to function as a group participant. If the group member chose not to participate that was one thing, but each member needed to be able to participate. The language of the group was English, so each member needed to be able to communicate in English. On one occasion this requirement was waived, and the client provided her own interpreter. The authors found that having a person involved with the group who was not actually a functioning member of the group was very disruptive. It was also revealed at subsequent meetings that other group members were not comfortable with this arrangement. The group was held during the daytime, so potential members who worked during daytime hours could not participate; this eliminated many potential members.

Participation of each potential group member was discussed at length by the client's case management team, which was composed of a physician, a nurse clinician, and a social worker. The recommendation of this team weighed heavily in the decision of whether to invite the older person with HIV/AIDS to participate in the group. Each case management team followed patients from their first clinic visit, through outpatient treatment, during any inpatient hospitalization, and on return to the clinic for outpatient follow-up. If a potential group member was under psychiatric care, the appropriateness of participation in a support–education group was discussed with the psychiatrist of record. The psychiatrist who was responsible for evaluating and treating patients in the clinic also provided supervision to the group cofacilitators.

Method

A proposal to establish a group was submitted to the administrators of the clinic. This proposal was accepted and then was submitted to the Department of Social Work for review and consideration. The Department of Social Work's established criteria for starting a group required some revisions in the initial focus and framework of the group. At that point, the focus and aim of the group were formally changed to include education as well as support. The group was then identified as a support–education group. Once the proposal was approved, the process of participant selection began.

Potential group members approved by the case management teams were sent an introductory letter that offered an invitation to join the group. The letter was carefully worded so as not to violate confidentiality as the authors did not know if the client would receive the letter directly. They also had no way of knowing if the client's HIV status had been shared with friends and family. The letter explained the intent of the group without mentioning HIV/AIDS. The letter spoke of giving people over the age of 50 who were members of the clinic an opportunity to explore issues important to them and their peers. This was done without specifically mentioning why these issues would be especially important to a client of the clinic. The letter closed by inviting people to telephone one of the cofacilitators for more information. When a potential group member who was stimulated by the letter made a phone inquiry, a number of questions and answers were exchanged.

This initial letter was followed by personal contact either by telephone or by connecting with the client during a regularly scheduled visit to the clinic. These attempts were met with various responses. Some clients could not be reached due to either incomplete telephone contact or a lack of interest on the part of the clients.

From the initial list, there were generated four subsequent lists of eligible group candidates. To the names on these lists, letters have been sent at intervals of approximately every 6 months. These lists generated names of previously unknown potential members, and introductory letters were sent to them. A different follow-up letter was sent to those people who were on the original list and had already received a letter. These letters were followed with another attempt at a telephone contact, by eliciting the help of the case management team in trying to reach the potential group member, or both. Included in each letter was a flyer announcing the time, date, and place of the group meeting. These flyers were generated with the same attention to privacy and confidentiality as in previous correspondence. They were also circulated throughout the hospital and posted in a number of clinical areas. The group was announced at a variety of meetings and colleagues were invited to refer clients for evaluation and consideration. Word of mouth was also used to notify others and announce the presence of the group.

COFACILITATORS' ISSUES

The cofacilitators in this project have their roots in different professional disciplines. One facilitator is a social worker with limited experience in group work but extensive experience working with the HIV-infected population. The other facilitator is a registered nurse with limited experience working with the HIV-infected population but extensive psychiatric, substance abuse, and group work and some geriatric experience. It was hoped that they could pool their knowledge and experiences and round out the services that they would provide to group members. The cofacilitators spoke openly about mutual and individual concerns and allowed for mistakes and issues of overlapping roles to be explored. They also found that enjoying each other's company and respecting each other's skills and attributes were beneficial to the process and outcome of this endeavor.

A major expectation that the cofacilitators had before starting the group was that the response would be overwhelming. They were concerned that they would either have to turn people away or consider starting a second group. These concerns proved to be unfounded. A major focus of their efforts has been on maintaining a core group. Much patience was needed for persisting in the early phases of the group. Adding new group members as people died or left is discussed later in this chapter.

There were various options for a meeting place. The group could meet in an area of the hospital other than one connected with the clinic, it could meet off-site, or it could meet in the clinic area. On consideration and out of concern for the confidential nature of the diagnosis, the members' comfort levels, and easy access, it was decided to have the group meet in an area of the hospital with which the members were familiar. The group started meeting in a conference room in the clinic area. As the demands for this space increased, it moved to another location. The group meets every other week for 1.5 hours in the morning. It was felt that this time would work out well because it would give people enough time to get to the session without the stress of an early morning trip to the hospital.

The results, observations, and notations described were based on contributions during initial in-depth interviews, group sessions, and one-on-one sessions. After each group meeting, the cofacilitators spent 30 minutes processing what had occurred during the group. Notes were made on each individual member as well as on the group as a whole.

The cofacilitators considered serving refreshments at each meeting; however, there were pros and cons to this issue. The use of food by members during group sessions can be seen as a coping mechanism. It can be used to deal with feelings instead of expressing them, and eating can interfere with self-disclosure by putting the focus on the experience of eating instead of on feelings and talking. However, the use of food to engage and facilitate process within a group is well-known. This particular age group finds it difficult to trust and self-disclose. Therefore, the authors decided to try any tool that could be used to facilitate trust and a sense of belonging. They learned that doughnuts, cookies, and cupcakes and tea and coffee can go a long way toward helping to establish a "safe place" for open, honest, and sometimes painful discussions.

INITIAL SESSIONS

Eight people attended the initial sessions; five (62.5%) were women; six (75%) had an AIDS diagnosis; and three (37%) had informed one or more significant persons of their HIV status. Women appeared to be more comfortable talking about their feelings and sharing them with others. When men were in attendance, women would allow the men to dominate and lead the discussion. These older women came from male-dominated backgrounds, and that pattern of interaction apparently carried over to their communication within the group. All of the original members were African American and came from the geographic area surrounding the hospital. The group eventually had another core member who was White and came from another area of the city.

Some of the group members were accompanied by companions or home health aides who waited in an area outside the group's meeting room. They became acquainted and formed their own informal support group, which was an unanticipated outgrowth of the planned group.

ISSUES OF CONCERN TO THE GROUP

One of the main issues discussed during the initial sessions was disclosure of HIV status to family members and significant others. Group members feared that they would be judged negatively by their adult children whom they thought saw them as role models. They feared feeling ashamed and guilty and that they would let their children down. One member was very surprised when she finally revealed her HIV status to her daughter. The young woman was accepting and concerned about her mother. The daughter was relieved because she had sensed that something was wrong but did not know what it was. Group members feared being stigmatized and rejected by those they depended on for support and love. They were already experiencing other losses as a result of growing older. They anticipated that once their HIV status was revealed they would suffer the loss of someone they loved and worried about feeling abandoned by the very people they needed most.

Another issue pertained to the fear of infecting others with HIV. One participant tearfully related her fear of having her grandson jump on her bed because she felt that he might contract the virus from her sheets. Another member was afraid to cook for her family over the holidays because she thought that she might give the virus to others if she touched the food. One woman canceled a vacation when she realized that she would have to share a bathroom with another person. She thought that she would pass the virus on to her friend by using the same facility. Through discussions with other group members and the cofacilitators, these irrational fears about how the virus is transmitted were corrected. The cofacilitators realized that members were, for the most part, under-informed and that they needed education, which needed to be reinforced periodically.

All of the women had become infected with HIV through a heterosexual relationship. Although the prevalent belief is that most older persons are infected through blood transfusions, the reality is that by 1990 10% of all AIDS cases in the over-50 population could be attributed to heterosexual transmission (Joslin, 1994). The women in the group were convinced they would have to remain "sexless" for the rest of their lives. They thought that this was the cause of their illness and that they would have to avoid sexual behaviors at all costs in the future. Because part of what the authors had initially set out to do was to educate, they invited a sex educator to one of the sessions. The subject was presented with sensitivity, and the group response was favorable. The members discovered there were many ways to express their sexuality and find warm, fulfilling relationships. They were also instructed on the use of condoms and ways of practicing safer sex.

Many discussions centered around present health status. Were the aches and pains they were feeling related to their progressing illness or just part of the aging process? Many times the cofacilitators were able to help them make distinctions among the various symptoms, but other times it was not clear. One woman had developed herpes zoster (shingles); although this is relatively common in older persons, she was worried that it was related to HIV. An older person can develop skin rashes due to increased skin sensitivity, but persons with AIDS can get similar rashes because of reactions to medications or as a result of a weakened immune system.

Medications were frequently discussed. Some members had very little understanding of what medications they were taking and what these medications were intended to do. Clarification was provided and encouragement given to them to ask more questions of their health care providers. Some of the current literature about new drugs was brought to the group, and the pros and cons of these new regimens were discussed. Members often compared the different medications they were taking, which helped to broaden the members' understanding of the wide variety of medications available. Repetition of information about various medications was needed during subsequent sessions to reinforce knowledge about this topic.

Videos were sometimes used as a springboard for discussions. Educational tapes produced by pharmaceutical companies, tapes of TV productions about AIDS topics, and full-length movies were shown. This approach did not generate much interaction. Some members stated that the videos made them sleepy and it was difficult to think clearly when they felt that way. Others simply said that they did not think the tapes were very interesting.

Frequent attempts were made to discuss the topics of death, dying, and end-of-life issues. Initially these attempts were met with interest and enthusiasm, but this soon faded. One person stated that when she became seriously ill and was convinced she was going to die soon, she would then tell her relatives and friends her diagnosis. The majority of the group members admitted that they knew they were going to die but did not want to dwell on the topic because it only made them feel worse. They did not feel that death loomed very large for them now, and they wanted to spend time concentrating on living each day to the fullest. They could talk more easily about the death of a close relative or friend and the meaning that had for them, but, not surprisingly, had some difficulty talking about their own deaths.

During the year and a half that the group has been meeting, four people who had attended the group at one time or another have died. The group decided to memorialize them with a prayer and the lighting of a candle. Discussion of the impact of these deaths on the remaining members has been addressed in small doses. It seems that this is all group members are capable of handling, but the cofacilitators revisit the topic periodically. They have discussed advance directives (discussed in detail in chapter 8) such as the health care proxy (a document that designates a person to make critical decisions for them if they become incapable of doing so) and the do-not-resuscitate form (a document indicating that they do not want any life-sustaining equipment used to prolong their life if there is no hope of recovery). During one of the sessions, some group members stated they would choose suicide if they knew there was no hope of recovery. They took the health care proxy home with them to think about whom they might wish to designate to act on their behalf. The cofacilitators constantly remind themselves to accept the individual group members as they are, to present topics and let them proceed at their own pace. This is difficult at times, especially regarding the topic of death, as the authors feel that it is important that group members face the fact of their own mortality.

Members are encouraged to bring memorabilia and photographs of themselves, family, and friends, which has generated some of the best discussions the group has had. Members seemed to look forward to telling their stories. According to Sherman and Peak (1991, p. 73), "It is important to emphasize for practice purposes that most reminiscence is good for enhancing mood and self esteem. On this basis alone, it should be continued and encouraged in programming." Individual group members seemed more relaxed as they spoke about the events and people who had been important to them. As one spoke, another could hardly wait to interject a similar experience. Studies have shown that life review can help prepare a person for death. If one can accept the past, then acceptance of death is possible. One person expressed relief over the fact that a family member passed away without knowing about her HIV status. She said she would have felt guilty and ashamed if this person had known.

The guilt and shame felt by members is a subject that is often addressed by the group. They admit that if they had cancer or heart disease they would not hesitate to tell others. They would be understood, accepted, and supported. Smoking and eating the wrong foods are risk behaviors that contribute to cancer and heart disease. Yet the risk behaviors that contribute to HIV infection carry with them, in some instances, moral judgments that evoke guilt and shame. This discussion highlighted the fact that an AIDS diagnosis still carries with it the fear of being shunned by the majority of today's society.

Often discussions centered around the members' means of coping with the illness. Besides the support of the group, which has become very important to them, most have a strong spiritual foundation on which they rely. Each one approaches spirituality in a different way. Its use as a coping mechanism is supported in literature written about older persons and their use of religion and spirituality. Koenig, George, and Siegler (1988) found that almost half of the older respondents in their study reported that religious attitudes or actions helped them deal with life's stressful events. Some group members rely on their own personal inner resources, and others find support in attending religious services and the sense of fellowship that they find there.

One woman finds that her work and social life help her deal with the stress of being HIV-infected. Keeping busy helps her keep her mind off her problems, and she feels that dwelling on problems only heightens her anxiety. Another woman stated that she just accepts the fact that she is HIV-infected and goes on with her life. She has explored many of the possibilities for alternative treatments and has decided to stay with the medical regimen. Both of these women believe that besides following the prescribed treatment regimen there is very little they can do to change the course of their illness. They both find strength in the serenity prayer: "God, grant me the serenity to accept the things I cannot change, courage to change the things I can, and the wisdom to know the difference." Another participant maintains a very hopeful attitude. He believes that a cure will be found. This attitude of hopefulness is supported in the literature. Tobin (1988) found in his study of older persons' preservation of self that hopefulness helps reduce a person's vulnerability to stress. Except for the mutual support of the group members themselves and the one woman who told her daughter, no one in the group has any individual with whom they can talk about their HIV/AIDS-related concerns.

Laughter can be heard during many of the group sessions. Smith's (1994) article talked about dying AIDS patients and their rights. One of these rights is the right to laugh. People need to face the realities of serious illness and death, but they also need to continue experiencing ordinary humor and laughter. For most group members, this has been an integral part of their lives. They share jokes. One woman finds humorous stories about growing older and makes copies to bring to the group. They are able to laugh at themselves and their idiosyncrasies. Sessions are often part sublime and part ridiculous. The cofacilitators have introduced imagery exercises using humorous themes. These exercises have proved very effective. Again, the cofacilitators try to assess the group's needs on any given day. Humor is sometimes appropriate and sometimes not.

GROUP MEMBERS' INTERACTIONS AND REACTIONS

It has been interesting to observe the interactions of the group members. Initially all attention was directed toward the cofacilitators, but as members became more comfortable, they began to talk directly to each other and question and advise each other. When a member does not come to a session, the group discusses what that person's absence means. The absent person is usually missed, and concerns are always expressed about the person's health. There is always the fear that the illness has caught up with someone. This is understandable as at least one group member died suddenly. Two members have become close friends and have been communicating with each other outside the group.

One male participant who attended only one session was a former drug user and was quite sick, although he did manage to get to the group session on his own. He was mentally confused and somewhat disruptive throughout the session. This changed the usual pattern of interaction among the group members. They found it difficult to respond to him and were unsure about how they should react. This gentleman finally left before the session ended, and the remaining members expressed relief. The group talked about their reactions to this incident. It was pointed out that sometimes people react to stress with assertive or combative behavior. Members were concerned that they too may eventually experience mental confusion. This event provided an opportunity to readdress some end-of-life issues and give further education on the progression of the disease. This one-time group participant died shortly after this event, and group members had mixed feelings about it. They expressed sorrow over his death and also had to admit that they had not liked him very much.

Besides this man, there have been other participants who came only once.

The brief attendance by some persons was puzzling to the core members. They spoke very little when asked about their concerns regarding the deaths or the nonreturn of other members. It appears that these incidents have been forgotten. The emotional impact of these events on the members is addressed in subsequent sessions.

Because the group's purposes are support and education, there was sometimes confusion. Although they had been told it was not a social gathering, some new members came thinking it was. Others thought it was strictly a group where you could learn about benefits. One man came assuming that food was served and he could get a meal. A few came for other reasons and remained.

EVALUATION AND FUTURE PLANS

After a year and a half, the authors reevaluated the group's progress. The members themselves were pleased, felt supported, and were coming to the group sessions on a regular basis. The cofacilitators felt satisfied to have provided this opportunity for support to a forgotten AIDS population. Programs that enhance and strengthen a person's social network may be as clinically significant as implementing a medical procedure (Harel, 1988).

There was more to be done. The group was opened to the community at large. Flyers were sent to neighboring hospitals and community centers, and ads were placed in periodicals whose distribution reached professionals working in the AIDS field. The response was not overwhelming, but several inquiries were made and an AIDS patient from another hospital became a regular member of the group. Efforts continue to recruit new members using the original methods.

Future plans for the group include incorporating relaxation techniques, more imagery exercises, and continuing education on the value of nutrition and exercise for maintaining health and strength. The authors will continue to look at their goals and redefine them as necessary. Are members being helped to review life experiences and reconcile relationships? Are they being encouraged to express feelings about past and present loss of health? Are they being assisted in improving self-image and finding meaning in their lives?

WHAT THE COFACILITATORS HAVE LEARNED FROM THE EXPERIENCE

The cofacilitators have learned much from forming and facilitating this group over the past 18 months. They came to the realization that the formation of a group such as this takes a long time, and they have learned about the advantages of collaboration between nursing and social work. Nursing focuses on the health care concerns and social work on the psychosocial and entitlement issues, although sometimes areas of expertise overlap. Cofacilitating has practical advantages too. When one of the cofacilitators cannot be at a group session, the other fills in. As the group members are familiar with both cofacilitators, this does not disrupt group process.

The greatest learning experience is what the group members themselves have taught the cofacilitators. Being able to share their roller coaster ride as they deal with HIV/AIDS has been a rich, rewarding experience. Each member brings something unique to the group. Soft-spoken, gentle Mrs. Z, who is 72 years old and has worked with infants all her life, brings a mother's warmth. She never forgets to inquire about concerns that others have spoken about in prior sessions. It is often difficult to get her to talk about her needs. Mrs. M., 68 years old, is even-tempered and steady. Her manner always has a calming effect on the group. She has an infectious laugh that starts with a small snicker and bursts into a raucous guffaw that starts everyone laughing. Mrs. L., 65 years old, is vivacious and energetic. She is realistic about the course of her illness but approaches each day with enthusiasm. She has a keen sense of humor. Mrs. G., 50, who died recently, was very ill and walked with a cane. However, she was always meticulously groomed and took great pride in the way she looked. She said that if she looked good she felt better. Mr. W., in his mid-50s, was feisty. He died recently, but kept himself alive on sheer willpower for the last few months of his life. There are others who are equally inspiring. The authors feel privileged to have known them all.

REFERENCES

Alcoholics Anonymous. (1939). *Alcoholics Anonymous. The story of how many thousands of men and women have recovered from alcoholism* (3rd ed.). New York: Alcoholics Anonymous World Services.

Betz, R. L., Wilbur, M. P., & Roberts-Wilbur, J. (1981). A structural blueprint for group facilitators: Three group modalities. *Personnel and Guidance Journal, 60*(1), 31–37.

Cerio, J. E. (1979). Structured experience with the educational growth group. *Personnel and Guidance Journal, 57*(8), 398–401.

Conway, P. (1988). Losses and grief in old age. *Social Casework, 69*(9), 541–549.

Dupon, M., Bismuth, M. J., Parneix, P., Morlat, P., & Malou, M. (1991). Human immunodeficiency virus infection in patients over 60 years of age: A cohort study of 31 patients followed-up at the Regional University Hospital Center of Bordeaux. *Review of Medicine Internal, 12*(6), 419–423.

Gallo, F. (1982). Effects of social support networks on the health of the elderly. *Social Work in Health Care, 8*(2), 65–74.

Green, L. (1990). *Community health.* St. Louis, MO: C.V. Mosby.

Harel, Z. (1988). Coping with extreme stress and aging. *Social Casework, 69*(9), 575–583.

Joslin, D. (1994). HIV/AIDS and older adults. *CAPCO Capsules, 2*(1), 1–4.

Koenig, H. G., George, L. K., & Siegler, I. C. (1988). The use of religion and other emotion regulating coping strategies among older adults. *Gerontologist, 28*(3), 303–310.

Layzell, S., & McCarthy, M. (1992). Community-based health services for people with HIV/AIDS: A review from a health service perspective. *AIDS Care, 4*(2), 203–215.

Sherman, E., & Peak, T. (1991). Patterns of reminiscence and the assessment of late life adjustment. *Journal of Gerontological Social Work, 16*(1/2), 59–74.

Smith, D. (1994). A "last rights" group for people with AIDS. *The Journal for Specialists in Group Work, 19*(1), 17–21.

Tobin, S. (1988). Preservation of self in old age. *Social Casework, 69*(9), 550–555.

Toseland, R., Sherman, E., & Bliven, S. (1981). The comparative effectiveness of two group work approaches for the development of mutual support groups among the elderly. *Social Work with Groups, 4*(1/2), 137–153.

Wallace, J. I., Paauw, D. S., & Spach, D. H. (1993). HIV infection in older patients: When to suspect the unexpected. *Geriatrics, 48*(6), 61–64, 69–70.

Chapter 6

The Older Gay Man

Gregory Anderson

DEFINING THE PROBLEM

Since the beginning of the worldwide AIDS epidemic in the early 1980s, when AIDS was perceived as a "gay disease," much has been written on the subject. Gay men and their sexual and psychosocial lives became the subject of hundreds of articles in the professional medical, public health, and mental health journals. As a body of research began to emerge along with recommendations for treatment, education, and prevention strategies and implications for public policy, it became apparent that research was still focusing on gay men under the age of 50 as they did represent the majority of cases in the early years of the epidemic.

As epidemiologists watched HIV infection spread into other populations—injecting drug users (IDUs) and their sexual partners, women, children, and blood product recipients—they failed to notice that a significant number of older people were becoming infected, getting sick, and dying from AIDS. Any discussion of AIDS and aging must apply the same scrutiny and professional rigor to older gay and bisexual men, who still compose approximately 67% of all geriatric AIDS cases in this country (Centers for Disease Control, 1993). In New York City, where the incidence of AIDS among gay men under 50 now consists of fewer than 50% of the total AIDS population, gay and bisexual men still account for 54% of all cases involving persons over 50 (New York City Department of Health, 1994). In New York City, the percentage of gay and bisexual men in the over-50 AIDS population has been declining in the past few years because of a dramatic increase in the number of older IDUs. Nonetheless, the actual numbers of older gay men with HIV/AIDS continues to grow. Unless society can commit itself to creating appropriate outreach, education, and prevention strategies targeted at older gay men, it can expect the numbers of new cases to increase throughout the 1990s and into the next millennium.

As the last two International Conferences on AIDS (Munich, Germany, in 1993 and Yokohama, Japan, in 1994) have shown, the thrust of scientific research has shifted dramatically to the development of treatments to prolong and enhance the quality of life for persons with AIDS (PWAs) in the absence of a cure or vaccine (Anderson, 1994). What is becoming increasingly clear is that many individuals infected with HIV in middle and late middle age will survive into older age with HIV. What researchers are learning now about older gay men and their capacity to cope and survive with HIV/AIDS will be invaluable to all health care and social service providers as the HIV/AIDS community ages.

IDENTIFYING AND SERVING THE POPULATION

There are serious problems in identifying and serving the population of older gay men with HIV/AIDS that have plagued service providers since the issue first came to attention in the late 1980s. The epidemic was nearing the end of its first decade, and many in the AIDS and aging networks were practicing their own brand of denial. The AIDS network of health and social service providers who were used to working with younger gay men were not looking for HIV disease in older gay men, and those in the aging network were similarly unwilling to imagine that older gay male clients might be at risk or already infected with HIV. The field of lesbian and gay gerontology, which is still very much in its infancy, has taught researchers a great deal about the lives of older gay men. The research of Kelly (1977), Kimmel (1978), and Berger (1977, 1982, 1984) identified the psychosocial issues, and a clearly defined culture of the older gay man in American society began to emerge. Organizations such as Senior Action in a Gay Environment (SAGE), a multiservice social service organization in New York City for older gay men and lesbians, were started to provide service to this population. The professional social work staff at SAGE had been providing case management services to homebound gay and lesbian elderly persons, as well as social and educational programs to mobile seniors, since the early 1980s. However, SAGE found itself quite unprepared for the first cases of HIV in its clientele in 1988. The development of SAGE's model AIDS and the Elderly program is discussed in greater detail later in this chapter as an example of how programming for older gay men with HIV/AIDS evolved. The following case example illustrates the denial that was prevalent among organizations and individuals at the time:

> A call came to the SAGE office from Darryl, an active member of the organization. His 55-year-old lover, Everett, was in the hospital and would be there over

the holidays. Everett was quite depressed and in need of some cheering up. Darryl was somewhat evasive about the nature of the hospitalization. It was decided that a hospital visit was indicated, and a social worker was assigned. The cause of the hospitalization turned out to be shingles, which is not uncommon in 55-year-old men. The social worker, who was quite familiar with HIV disease, suspected immediately that Everett's shingles were HIV-related. Everett admitted to the social worker that this was the case. Darryl and Everett were both extremely agitated during the hospital visit. Everett was incredulous and said that he had no idea how he could have become infected. His primary concern was that no one find out about his HIV status. He was concerned about his employer and about his mentally ill sister with whom he shared an apartment. The social worker arranged for two of SAGE's volunteer Friendly Visitors to help keep Everett company over the holidays and offer Darryl some respite. A treatment plan was initiated that involved weekly visits by the social worker to Everett's home following the hospitalization to begin helping him sort through his options while coming to some acceptance of his change in health.

In the months following Everett's initial contact with SAGE, a debate developed over the meaning of his illness and the possibility of changing the agency's mandate to serve older gay men with AIDS. Investigations by the agency's clinical director led staff to believe that Everett was not an isolated case and that other AIDS agencies were beginning to see cases in older gay men. The idea of a SAGE program for older men with HIV/AIDS was presented to the executive director, who flatly rejected the idea. She felt there was little evidence to support the need for such a program. It was her contention that seniors with HIV/AIDS could be better served by existing programs such as the Gay Men's Health Crisis. A compelling argument was put forward by the executive director and by the board of directors that a program for HIV/AIDS would only serve to dilute the organization's original mission. She made it clear that SAGE was not going to become an AIDS organization.

It was only because of the clinical director's persistence that a pilot program entitled AIDS and the Elderly was launched. She surmised that the isolation traditionally experienced by older gay men could only be exacerbated by HIV/AIDS and that an outreach effort could possibly reveal the extent of the problem. With the help of a volunteer facilitator, a new support group for HIV-positive men over the age of 50 was advertised; 35 men showed up for the first meeting on a hot August evening. Not surprisingly, that large turnout at SAGE's first event raised more questions than it answered. Was there really a large, undiscovered population of older gay men with HIV/AIDS? If so, why were they not being served by other AIDS organizations? SAGE would soon find out that there was a great discrepancy between the public and professional perception of HIV/AIDS demographics and the extent of its incidence in the older gay community. To begin to understand why HIV had remained a secret for so long in the older gay community, it is necessary to return to knowledge of gay and lesbian gerontology and to put HIV/AIDS into a historical context.

THE CULTURE OF THE OLDER GAY MAN

To understand how an individual responds to a chronic or terminal illness, one is often aided by research that is done with a particular group of individuals who are living with that condition. Much has been written on gay men and their psychological response to HIV/AIDS, but little has, been written on the cohort of older gay men. The best one can do in this situation is to apply what has been learned from gay gerontological studies to knowledge about younger gay men and HIV/AIDS. Examples from the author's clinical practice with older gay men with HIV/AIDS over the past 6 years are used to clarify what has been inferred. To understand how older gay men are responding to HIV/AIDS, it is important to put their psychosocial development into a historical context. The older gay man today was socialized in the late 1920s, 1930s, and 1940s in what is now known to have been a time of open hostility toward gay and lesbian people. It has subsequently been learned that periods of increased tolerance preceded this time, most notably the period from the 1890s to the 1920s, when a well-defined and quite open gay male culture emerged in New York City (Chauncey, 1994). For the older gay man of today, though, the years of early socialization were a time of extreme condemnation from the church, medicine, psychiatry, the military, and the law (Berger, 1980). Few dissenting voices were raised during this period, and the gay movement was very much underground and out of reach of most gay men. It was not until the mid-1960s that the professional silence on the subject was broken. The research by Hooker (1965) and others on psychologically well-adjusted gay men would eventually lead the mental health community to a drastic rethinking of its position on homosexuality as a pathological condition. By this time, however, the damage to today's gay seniors had already been done. By the time of the Stonewall rebellion in 1969 and the birth of today's gay civil rights movement, many gay men had already learned to survive by living double lives, and "the closet" had become the norm for a generation. By learning to "pass" in straight society, most accomplished the task of managing a discreditable identity (Goffman, 1963). However, they internalized society's negative assessments of homosexuality along the way. Low self-esteem, poor self-image, and depression were some of the lasting consequences for a generation of gay men. Why many survived the same harsh societal treatment with sound mental health in later life is the subject of the current research in gay and lesbian gerontology. These themes are returned to as the interplay of HIV/AIDS and the coping mechanisms of this generation of gay men is explored.

The societal institutions that assist in times of crisis caused by chronic or terminal illness are the very institutions that have caused conflict for today's older gay men. Treated by the medical and psychiatric communities as individuals in need of a "cure" for their homosexuality, older gay men often carry with them a deep-seated mistrust of health professionals (Passer, 1988). Labeled *sinners* and excluded from religious life in their communities of origin, they are mistrustful of spiritual interventions. Archaic sodomy laws in this country have been enforced unequally against gay men, and many in this generation have served time in prison for morals charges that damaged their ability to interact with the legal and law enforcement communities. Also, despite the fact that more than 2 million gay men and lesbians served in the armed forces in World War II (Berube, 1990), those most in need of veterans' services are categorically denied them because of dishonorable discharges. Many older gay men have built and relied on alternative professional support networks, but many, especially those living with HIV/AIDS, continue to be victimized by societal injustice. As the ramifications of HIV/AIDS on the lives of older gay men begin to be explored, it is important to recognize that the cohort of older gay men is incredibly diverse. Many of them married to conform to society's standards, raised families, and are now grandparents and great-grandparents, and many others found lifetime partners of the same sex. They worked in the public and private sectors, and although many did migrate to larger cities to escape persecution within their families and communities of origin, older gay men thrive in every small town and rural community in the United States. Many choose, though, to remain invisible, and that choice is based on a realistic appraisal of past and present prejudice against gay people in this society. This self-imposed isolation separates these men from the larger gay and lesbian community and from the larger HIV/AIDS community when they become infected. Discussion in this chapter is confined primarily to the urban older gay man with HIV/AIDS.

RISK FACTORS FOR THE OLDER GAY MAN

Sexual Practice

Because the highest risk behavior for HIV transmission for older gay men remains sexual contact (Stall & Catania, 1994), it is important to understand how and why this cohort puts itself at risk. Earlier studies revealed valuable information about the sexual practices of older gay men. Weinberg and Williams (1974) found that gay men over 45 visited gay bars less often and had greater difficulty finding sexual partners than younger gay men, which made them less likely to contract the virus through sexual contact. However, older gay men appear to have more difficulty negotiating the change to safer sex practices (Anderson, 1994). During their adolescence and early and middle adulthood, this generation of men had little to fear from unprotected sex other than easily treatable sexually transmitted diseases. Many are finding it difficult to incorporate safer sex practices into their sexual repertoire. Although older gay men are quite knowledgeable about HIV transmission and are concerned about the epidemic (Kooperman, 1994), many express the sentiments of a 67-year-old client who said, "Our people don't use condoms." The older gay man who may have lived alone all his life or who may have suffered the loss of a lifetime partner may increasingly rely on hustlers for sexual companionship.

Substance Abuse

In New York City and other places in the United States where the HIV epidemic has intersected with the drug epidemic, the sexual marketplace has become a place of compromise. Older men and younger hustlers find themselves bargaining away safer sex measures in the negotiating process. This may be especially true when alcohol or drugs are used by both men as a prelude to a sexual encounter. It has long been established that gay men and lesbians have significantly higher rates of alcoholism than the general population (Zehner & Lewis, 1984) and that adherence to safer sex practices is more difficult when the participants are impaired through the use of alcohol or drugs (Odets, 1994).

Injecting Drug Use

It is also difficult to track the population of older IDUs by sexual orientation; however, in New York City the number of older HIV-infected IDUs reporting sex with men is quite small (approximately 2% of the total over-50 AIDS population; New York City Department of Health, 1994).

High-Risk Behavior

The older gay man who may have closeted himself in a traditional marriage may be particularly vulnerable to HIV infection, as he may need to rely more on anonymous encounters or paid hustlers for homosexual contact. It is assumed that high-risk sexual behavior is more prevalent in these settings and that the fear of bringing a sexually transmitted disease back to the home is often not sufficient to steer these men toward safer behavior. Catania, Turner, Kegeles, et al. (1989) suggested that the more closeted a man is, the less likely he is to have internalized the changing sexual mores of the gay community and to be reducing high-risk sexual activity as a result of exposure to safer sex education.

Venereal Disease

Berger (1977), in a study of older gay men, found high levels of sexual activity and corresponding high levels of venereal infection. He found men who had been repeatedly exposed and treated for sexually transmitted diseases in their adult lives. An extensive history of venereal infection may correlate with a higher HIV transmission risk. Martin and Vance (1984) discussed the vulnerability of an individual to infection as a function of the immune system's competence and responsiveness. It is known that older adults experience a normal decline in immune response, but it is not known if this makes the older gay man with a history of venereal infection more vulnerable to HIV infection. This is certainly an area for needed research.

Blood Transfusion

Older adults are the greatest recipients of blood products in this country. As discussed earlier in this book, before the development in 1985 of a blood test to screen the blood supply for HIV antibody, many older Americans were infected. The morbidity rate for this group was very high, and most died within a few years of infection. There are very few data on the breakdown of this population by sexual orientation, and one can only assume that a percentage of this group consisted of gay men.

OLDER GAY MEN
AND HEALTH CARE PROVIDERS

There is much discussion in the AIDS and aging networks concerning the role of the health care provider and the older adult. Many older gay men have never disclosed their sexual orientation to their health care providers. Older gay men, unwilling or unable to come out to their physicians, often collude with their medical practitioners, who themselves are unable to discuss the behavior of sexual minorities. It is common practice in the older gay male community to see a variety of health care providers. An older gay man may have a long-term relationship with a general practitioner or an internist with whom he is closeted and a gay doctor whom he may see only for the treatment of venereal infections. This fragmentation of health care can have disastrous consequences in the presence of HIV/AIDS when one care provider is accorded only limited access to the full medical picture. As was seen in chapter 3, the possibility of misdiagnosis of HIV infection is great if the care provider sees the patient as being at low risk for HIV. Although the number of openly gay physicians has increased dramatically in the past 20 years, it may still be difficult for the generation of older gay men to come out to a health professional. The stigma of being seen entering or leaving the office of a known gay physician may be too much for the older gay man who has devoted tremendous energy to preserving his secret. As long as the wall of silence between older gay men and their health care providers remains in place, misinformation rules and the risk of undiagnosed HIV infection remains high. It is becoming increasingly clear that the HIV prevention message is not reaching older adults, including older gay men. All possible means of providing relevant safer sex information to older gay men must be explored. Older gay men who have managed their sexual lives with utmost discretion may still exhibit some confusion about the distinction between discretion and safer sex. A 70-year-old sexually active client who was asked if he was using a condom every time replied, "Oh, you have nothing to fear. I've always been discrete." The answer to this question was actually "no," but the client remained adamant in his conviction because his new partner was from a "good family." Geriatricians play a vital role in the medical education of their older patients (Lomax, 1980). Unfortunately, most physicians today have difficulty taking complete sexual histories of their patients, especially of patients much older than themselves. Only in the past 20 years have U.S. medical schools begun to provide students with even rudimentary sex education. It will be some time before geriatricians and other health care providers can be expected to convey safer sex information that will be necessary to lower the risk of HIV infection in older gay men.

LIVING WITH HIV/AIDS

Fear of HIV/AIDS is rampant in society and, for persons who have engaged in high-risk behaviors, the fear of being tested for HIV antibody can be overwhelming. Many older gay men refuse to be tested. This generation has seen AIDS emerge in the early 1980s as a mysterious "gay cancer," become gay-related immune disorder, and finally become a full-fledged epidemic. Many have experienced profound personal loss. With little hope for a cure or a vaccine in the near future, they see an AIDS diagnosis as a death sentence. The crisis of diagnosis may be especially difficult for older gay men who have managed a closeted way of dealing with their homosexuality throughout their adult lives. The more closeted the older gay man, the more likely is a diagnosis of HIV seropositivity to shatter the man's social system. Cates, Graham, Boeglin, and Tielker (1990) discussed the anger, sense of betrayal, and personal inadequacy that a wife can experience when she discovers that her husband of many years and the father of her children is not only gay but HIV-positive. The following case example illustrates this kind of family disruption:

> Edward is a 60-year-old physician who suffered a stroke. At the time of his hospitalization it was apparent to his primary physician that he was immune-suppressed. He was tested for HIV and diagnosed seropositive. His physician informed his wife and two adult children, and Edward was forced to discuss his sexual history with men with them. His wife immediately sued for divorce and his children abandoned him. He became severely depressed. He suffered from mild ataxia, a moderate speech impediment, and had difficulty walking. His adult son, who had assumed his father's power of attorney, found him an apartment, hired home health attendants, and gave him a small allowance, but wished no further contact with him. Edward was cut off from his family as well as his professional associates and became extremely isolated. In a very short amount of time he had gone from being a highly respected and wealthy professional with a family to a man who was virtually broke, ill, and in the care of strangers.

Edward's may be an extreme case, but for the closeted older gay man, it is not an unusual one. Because older gay men are often cut off from the kinds of social supports that younger gay men have when they are diagnosed, they often experience profound depression. The reactions to HIV diagnosis of older gay men, many of whom have experienced a lifetime of depressive symptomatology, are generally poor. If one can measure an individual's movement from denial and depression to acceptance of HIV/AIDS, as described by Kübler-Ross (1987), one can begin to see how older gay men differ from the general AIDS population.

Denial

To date there has been no significant research to measure the response of older gay men to an AIDS diagnosis. Researchers know from literature on breast cancer that women who take an active interest in their illness and in health promotion, who join support groups, and who seek out psychotherapy have a better prognosis and a better psychological adaptation to the processes of illness and recovery (Greer, Morris, & Pettingale, 1979; Holland & Mastrovito, 1980).

Researchers also know that younger gay men with HIV/AIDS are more likely to be proactive in their treatment and to be politically active in the AIDS movement. It is the experience at SAGE that older gay men, however, experience difficulty even in following through on referrals to support groups and other support services. Three out of four referrals to SAGE's AIDS and the Elderly program are not followed up by the client. This is seen now as older gay men adding another bolt to the closet door and further isolating themselves as a result of their illness (Anderson, 1991). Denial occurs in many forms among older gay men with HIV/AIDS. The overwhelming anxiety experienced by most individuals on learning they have a life-threatening illness can bring on a variety of denial-based defensive responses. The early, almost shut-down response seen in many older gay men is one of complete denial: "I don't have AIDS, I'm only HIV-positive, and who knows what that means anyway. Doctors don't really know what that means." SAGE often sees the man who goes home from his first AIDS-related hospitalization, sits in front of the TV, "forgets" to take his medication, and "forgets" to follow up on clinic appointments or support group referrals. SAGE sees older gay men in extraordinary situations cope with the presence of HIV/AIDS, trying to maintain order and regularity in a life seemingly made chaotic and unmanageable by an HIV/AIDS diagnosis.

> Frederick is a 62-year-old gay male who shares a large apartment in New York City with his 67-year-old brother and his 91-year-old mother. Frederick was diagnosed with HIV but was without symptoms for almost 2 years. He continued to work full time as a hairdresser, which was work that he enjoyed, brought him a great deal of validation, and formed the locus of his support network. Two years later, he was diagnosed with Kaposi's sarcoma and began interferon treatments three times weekly. At that time Frederick's mother still maintained the household, but many of the responsibilities were beginning to fall on Frederick. His older brother was ill with terminal liver cancer, a subject that caused everyone in the household great concern. At the time of his HIV diagnosis Frederick swore to himself that no one in the family would learn of his condition. His older brother was aware of his sexual orientation, but it was never discussed. To Frederick's knowledge, his mother was unaware that he was gay. Frederick's reaction to interferon was not atypical. He would leave the beauty shop mid-afternoon for his treatment and be home by 5:00 p.m. By early evening he would develop flulike symptoms, sometimes quite severe, and retreat to his private bathroom to lie on the cold floor between bouts of vomiting. This went on for several weeks during the treatment. The members of Frederick's support group for HIV-positive gay men over 50 encouraged him to talk about what it felt like to have to keep his illness secret and to consider telling his family what was wrong. Frederick was adamant and eventually dropped out of the group when the peer pressure became too great.

Guilt, Resignation, and Withdrawal

Along with denial and depression, SAGE sees older gay men displaying a great deal of guilt and resignation. "I have nothing to complain about. I've had a full life. It's these young kids with their whole lives ahead of them that I feel sorry for. It makes me feel guilty taking up the doctor's time," one older man with AIDS said. Whether this kind of self-effacing behavior is the product of a lifetime in the closet or a normative working through of developmental issues (Lavick, 1994), it is difficult for these men to believe in any kind of future.

Perhaps the most brutal manifestation of resignation is displayed by many of these men: "Look at the life I've led. I've gotten exactly what I deserve." These men, for whom there were few opportunities to establish long-term relationships, have so fully internalized society's negative assessments of their sexual behavior that they find it difficult to believe that HIV is just a virus. For many of them, it is almost a message from God about a life ill spent. It is important to remember that the emotional and psychological responses to HIV/AIDS in the cohort of older gay men fall along a continuum. As this chapter looks at intervention models for this population, it examines the resilient and more adaptive responses of a healthier portion of the population.

It is generally understood that the HIV/AIDS epidemic has brought about enormous changes in the relationship patterns and sexual behavior of all gay men (Morin, Charles, & Malyon, 1984). For older gay men who may never have developed the skills for interpersonal relations or who may have lost a lifetime partner, the future appears bleak. In the presence of HIV/AIDS, many seem unwilling or unable to explore the possibility of a new primary relationship or even new nonsexual friendships. It is a common reaction for older gay men with HIV/AIDS to withdraw from the arena of relationships because the future, or what is perceived to be left of it, is more easily managed alone. Although some clinicians who work with HIV-positive gay men report that their clients display increased sexual activity and sexual compulsivity following diagnosis, the opposite seems to be true of older gay men. Older gay men report a dramatic loss of interest in sex and in some cases complete impotence. There seem to be two primary causal factors: a sense of contamination that makes them feel unattractive and afraid of contaminating others (despite a complete or partial awareness of current guidelines for safer sex) and a dramatically reduced libido, possibly caused by the antiretroviral and prophylactic medications and the medications commonly used by older men to treat hypertension, heart disease, diabetes, and prostate disease. This dual loss of interest in interpersonal relations and loss of interest or ability in sexual relations only compounds the isolation often seen in older gay men with HIV/AIDS. Whether an individual reacts to an HIV diagnosis with denial and isolation or is able to move through these feelings to some kind of acceptance depends on many premorbid factors. The process will be accelerated for older adults because older adults progress to end-stage AIDS faster than younger adults (Ship, Wolff, & Selik, 1991). It is unclear whether this is due to normal immune decline in older adults, to delayed diagnosis, or to some other factor. For the older gay man, quality-of-life issues after diagnosis are both quantitative and qualitative.

INTERVENTIONS

The SAGE Model

Several issues have emerged for AIDS and aging health and social service providers since it was acknowledged that older adults with HIV/AIDS were in need of service. Questions arose as to how to best serve the population of older gay men. This section explores intervention models and intervention alternatives. The SAGE model for serving older gay men with HIV/AIDS grew out of a demonstrated need for services specifically tailored to this subpopulation of the HIV/AIDS community. Older gay men were not being adequately treated by traditional aging service providers or by the community of HIV/AIDS service providers. The SAGE model, since its inception, has sought to serve this population by providing a supportive agency environment staffed by clinicians trained and experienced in gay and lesbian gerontology and in state-of-the-art HIV/AIDS treatment.

Involvement with the SAGE program begins with a comprehensive needs assessment and an introduction to the services provided. For many older gay men, this may be their first opportunity to open up and discuss feelings about HIV/AIDS with another human being. This can be an overwhelming and emotionally charged experience. The first layer of denial may be broken through, and some men are never seen again. Any discussion of one's health status and the entitlements, benefits, and programs available to a person with HIV/AIDS brings up issues of life expectancy and mortality. This first level of intervention may need to be handled with extreme sensitivity as many of these men are not prepared to live with HIV/AIDS, only to die from it.

SAGE Plus

Older gay men with HIV/AIDS often bring to SAGE a sense of estrangement not only from their peers but from their illness as well. The support groups for HIV-positive men over 50, known as SAGE Plus groups, provide men with an opportunity to share their experiences with HIV disease in an age-appropriate context. The groups, the first of which began in August 1989, are closed, ongoing groups that are facilitated by one or two SAGE group workers. The members of the group at any given time encompass the newly diagnosed to long-term survivors, which has presented real challenges to group cohesion (Burke, Coddington, Bakeman, & Clance, 1994). Many newly diagnosed men find it extremely painful to observe the disease process at close range as it takes its toll on the less healthy members. These men often drop out, only to return to the group after their first opportunistic infection and hospitalization. The group facilitators have had to be flexible by allowing group members to develop their own rules about participation and commitment. Some men are simply not able to manage the stress of weekly attendance. The group members fluctuate in their ability to handle difficult subjects and emotions and may spend a great deal of the group's time engaging in reminiscence and gossip.

In a group whose members encompass the spectrum of HIV disease, there is the possibility for much positive mentoring. Older men who may be cut off from the rest of the gay community rely on each other in the group setting for the exchange of medical information, treatment options, entitlements, and other supportive services. The more long-term members of the group can be positive role models for the newly diagnosed, who may still be overwhelmed with fear and feelings of hopelessness. Older gay men who might be expected to be rigid adherents to Western medicine can learn from each other the myriad possibilities of alternative therapies. The group process can help older gay men find a healthier balance between an obsessive fear of death and a need to engage in magical denial of the realities of their illness (Getzel & Mahony, 1990).

Caregiver support. An HIV diagnosis can bring on profound changes in a long-term relationship or in any nontraditional family unit. Support For You, a caregivers' support group, allows longtime partners, friends, and others caring for an older PWA to share their experiences in this difficult role. Caregivers often have the same needs and concerns as the PWA—fear of contagion, fear of death, shame, guilt, and stigma—but are often neglected by the need to mobilize support for the person who is ill (Greif & Porembski, 1989). The older couple may be quite isolated, having already lost the support of family and friends due to illness and death, and the presence of HIV/AIDS in one or both partners can be further isolating. It is not uncommon for both partners in a couple to be HIV-positive, with the healthier of the two caring for the other.

SAGE has quite successfully integrated caregivers and the bereaved into Support For You. Group members enter the groups as caregivers and remain to work through the grieving process. Newcomers are welcomed and supported through the caregiving process while observing the pain and subsequent healing of bereavement. By the time of the partner's death from HIV/AIDS, the caregiver is bonded to the group and ready to begin the work of accepting the loss. In both the SAGE Plus and the Support For You groups, there is the added element of socialization with peers. Members of the groups form informal alliances outside of the group, provide telephone reassurance to one another, visit one another in the hospital, and socialize between regularly scheduled meetings. The organization has had less success, unfortunately, in integrating members of SAGE Plus into social events regularly scheduled for the SAGE membership at large. The older HIV-positive members of SAGE have not always felt particularly welcome at larger social events. More than one member has reported back to the support group that he was ostracized for being "the one with AIDS."

Other alternatives. Certain older gay men with HIV/AIDS do not do well in support groups, and for them SAGE offers individual treatment, including psychiatric and psychopharmacological intervention when necessary. Men who are too closeted about their HIV status or who are too uncomfortable in group settings still do well in individual therapy. Older gay men with sufficient ego strength and coping skills do manage their illness without much outside intervention. For them, diagnosis can be a crystallizing event, one that brings a focus to their lives and a determination to live fully and usefully during the time they have left. These individuals may use the treatment services at SAGE to work on the goals of traditional psychotherapy, such as the resolution of intrapsychic conflict or the developmental issues of later life. One client reported that he had never realized his own creative potential until he was diagnosed. On that day he realized he'd "better get crackin' and live."

Outreach and advocacy. The clinical staff at SAGE has acknowledged that outreach efforts must include the mainstream aging network and other HIV/AIDS service providers. Since the beginning of the gay and lesbian social service movement in the 1970s, the question of whether to use mainstream agencies has been debated. Some older gay men with HIV/AIDS may be more comfortable receiving service in mainstream aging organizations. SAGE's program of public and professional education now administers a grant from the Burden Foundation in New York City to train aging service providers on issues of gay and lesbian gerontology and on intervention strategies with gay men with HIV/AIDS. It is clear that this population must always have choices around disclosure of sexual orientation and HIV status and the freedom to choose nongay settings to receive service. It is equally important for other AIDS health and social service providers to become sensitive to the needs of their older gay male clients. This population may always need to rely on the larger AIDS organizations, such as the Gay Men's Health Crisis, for meals and nutritional services, certain entitlement services, and legal services. SAGE has extended itself to the AIDS network to begin a dialogue about the older gay man in an intergenerational setting. Likewise, the older gay man with HIV/AIDS may have unique needs and problems in institutional settings. Outreach to long-term care facilities (nursing homes, hospitals, and hospices) will be equally important to alert these institutions to the psychosocial issues of the population.

SUMMARY

As understanding of the unique aspects of HIV/AIDS in the older gay male population grows, it will be important to share expertise and to advocate for the population. Creating awareness in the gay and lesbian health and social service network and in the gerontological community is a priority. In the past few years, the American Society on Aging and the Gerontological Society of America have made AIDS and aging a priority in their publications and at national conferences. Likewise, the National Lesbian and Gay Health Association is giving similar attention to the issue. The ultimate goal must always be toward the improvement of care for the older individual with HIV/AIDS and the development of sound education and prevention strategies.

REFERENCES

Anderson, G. (1991, September). *HIV/AIDS line.* (Available from HIV/AIDS Services, Room 618, 325 Loyola Ave., New Orleans, LA 70112).

Anderson, G. (1994). HIV prevention and older people. *SIECUS Report, 23*(2), 18–20.

Berger, R. (1977). Report on a community-based venereal clinic for homosexual men. *Journal of Sex Research, 13,* 54–62.

Berger, R. M. (1980). Psychological adaptation of the older homosexual male. *Journal of Homosexuality, 5,* 161–175.

Berger, R. (1982). The unseen minority. Older gays and lesbians. *Social Work, 27,* 236–241.

Berger, R. M. (1984). The realities of gay and lesbian aging. *Social Work, 29,* 57–62.

Berube, A. (1990). *Coming out under fire.* New York: Free Press.

Burke, J. M., Coddington, D., Bakeman, R., & Clance, P. R. (1994). Inclusion and exclusion in HIV support groups. *Journal of Gay & Lesbian Psychotherapy, 2,* 121–131.

Catania, J., Turner, H., Kegeles, S., Stall, R., Pollack, L., & Coates, T. (1989). Older Americans and AIDS: Transmission prevention research needs. *The Gerontologist, 29,* 373–381.

Cates, J. A., Graham, L. L., Boeglin, D., & Tielker, S. (1990, April). The effect of AIDS on the family system. *The Journal of Contemporary Human Services,* 195–201.

Centers for Disease Control. (1993, October). U.S. AIDS cases through September 1993. *HIV/AIDS Surveillance Report, 5*(3).

Chauncey, G. (1994). *Gay New York: Gender, urban culture, and the making of the gay male world 1890–1940.* New York: Basic Books.

Getzel, G. S., & Mahony, K. F. (1990). Confronting human finitude: Group work with people with AIDS. *Journal of Gay & Lesbian Psychotherapy, 1,* 105–119.

Goffman, E. (1963). *Stigma: Notes on the management of spoiled identity.* Englewood Cliffs, NJ: Prentice-Hall.

Greer, S., Morris, T. E., & Pettingale, K. W. (1979). Psychological response to breast cancer: Effect on outcome. *Lancet, 2,* 785–787.

Greif, G. L., & Porembski, E. (1989). Implications for therapy with significant others of persons with AIDS. *Journal of Gay & Lesbian Psychotherapy, 1,* 79–86.

Holland, J. C., & Mastrovito, R. (1980). Psychologic adaption to breast cancer. *Cancer, 46,* 1045–1052.

Hooker, E. (1965). Male homosexuals and their worlds. In J. Marmor (Ed.), *Sexual inversion* (pp. 83–107). New York: Basic Books.

Kelly, J. (1977). The aging male homosexual: Myth and reality. *The Gerontologist, 17,* 328–332.

Kimmel, D. C. (1978). Adult development and aging: A gay perspective. *Journal of Social Issues, 34*(3), 113–131.

Kooperman, L. (1994). *A survey of gay and bisexual men age 50 and over.* Unpublished manuscript.

Kübler-Ross, E. (1987). *AIDS: The ultimate challenge.* New York: Collier Books.

Lavick, J. (1994). *Psychosocial considerations of HIV infection in the older adult.* Unpublished manuscript.

Lomax, J. (1980). Social support in geriatric education. *Family Medicine Teacher, 12*(6), 9–12.

Martin, J. L., & Vance, C. S. (1984). Behavioral and psychological factors in AIDS. *American Psychologist, 39,* 1303–1307.

Morin, S. F., Charles, K. A., & Malyon, A. K. (1984). The psychological impact of AIDS on gay men. *American Psychologist, 39,* 1288–1293.

New York City Department of Health. (1994, July). *AIDS surveillance update.* New York: New York City Department of Health.

Odets, W. (1994) AIDS education and harm reduction for gay men: Psychological approaches for the 21st century. *AIDS & Public Policy Journal, 9*(1), 3–15.

Passer, D. (1988). The gay physician: Out of the closet. In M. Shernoff & W. A. Scott (Eds.), *The sourcebook on lesbian/gay health care* (pp. 41–44). Washington, DC: National Lesbian/Gay Health Foundation.

Ship, J. A., Wolff, A., & Selik, R. A. (1991). Epidemiology of acquired immune deficiency syndrome in persons age 50 years or older. *Journal of Acquired Immune Deficiency Syndrome, 4*(1), 84–88.

Stall, R., & Catania, J. (1994). AIDS risk behavior among late middle-aged and elderly Americans. *Archives of Internal Medicine, 154,* 57–63.

Weinberg, M. S., & Williams, C. (1974). *Male homosexuals.* New York: Oxford University Press.

Zehner, M. A., & Lewis, J. (1984). Homosexuality and alcoholism: Social and developmental perspectives. In R. Schoenberg & R. S. Goldberg (Eds.), *Homosexuality and social work* (pp. 75–86). New York: Haworth Press.

Chapter 7

Long-Term Care

Ann Wyatt

As people are living longer because of improvements in diagnosis and treatment, AIDS has increasingly taken on some of the characteristics of a chronic disease. Living with AIDS can now include not only episodes of acute illness but also periods of time with few or no symptoms at all. Most of the time, however, living with AIDS, like natural aging, also means living for extended periods of time with the symptoms of a variety of health care problems. This often means that in addition to treatment, help with various activities of daily living is also needed. For this reason, long-term care programs are coming to play an ever more prominent role in the care of people with AIDS.

Essentially, long-term care refers to personal care and other health and social services needed to compensate for a person's impairments in functioning; the focus is more on how one lives with illness than on the illness itself (Kane & Kane, 1987).

Initially, most AIDS care was provided in acute care hospitals, but now it is much more common for people with HIV/AIDS to receive care on an outpatient basis, and quite sophisticated treatments are provided at home, as well as in nursing homes, hospices, and various other settings. There is, however, tremendous variation in the availability of these long-term care services. Both the kind and the extent of service available depends on where you live; whether you have friends or family able to help with your care; whether you have health insurance, and if you do, on the type; on your financial resources; and in some cases, on whether you are over 65 years of age.

This variation in the availability of services is essentially the product of a health care system that is disorganized and fragmented. For people with chronic illnesses who are dependent on these services for the daily conduct of their lives, such disorganization and fragmentation is particularly devastating. The Robert Wood Johnson Foundation (1994) recently completed a cycle of grants to providers of AIDS care across the country and concluded that the U.S. health care system is not organized to deal with the complex needs of people with chronic health problems. As a result, the foundation changed its approach by moving away from specific chronic disease categories and more toward tackling systemic problems in chronic disease care.

Related to the issue of fragmentation of services is the question of the extent to which AIDS-specific services should be organized separately within the overall health care system. When AIDS was first identified, the fact that it was new, unpredictable, and extremely complicated meant that services tended to be organized separately not only because of the stigma attached to the disease but also because it was a way of focusing fairly limited medical expertise and of ensuring appropriate and adequate care. Now that the HIV/AIDS epidemic is well into its second decade, there has been some greater integration of AIDS services within the health care system in general. Whether services should be integrated or AIDS-specific, and under what circumstances, has implications for long-term care.

Older people may face difficulties in receiving adequate or appropriate HIV/AIDS education and diagnostic services because of the public's perception that older people are not sexually active or that they are not likely to get AIDS. However, the question of whether older people with HIV/AIDS have sufficient access to AIDS-specific long-term care services is a different one. Nursing homes have traditionally been sources of skilled nursing and custodial care for frail elderly and disabled people who have functional impairments (Linsk, Cich, & Cianfrani, 1993). The long-term care system has had to make adjustments for AIDS patients who are often younger, and most AIDS-specific long-term care programs tend to be geared toward younger people. This does not mean older people are not welcome in these programs, or that they cannot find what they need. Some older people with AIDS may have available, and they may choose, traditional long-term care programs geared to older people. Most will probably not have such a choice, whereas some may in fact prefer AIDS-specific programs. There are also older people using a wide variety of aging services who have chosen not to disclose the fact that they have AIDS. In either type of long-term setting, however, there is the potential for older people to feel isolated. In traditional settings, they may feel the loneliness of facing a disease with such stigma attached to it, whereas in AIDS-specific settings they may simply lack the company of other older people.

Finally, it must be kept in mind that the whole range of long-term care services, including housing, tends to work interdependently: The relative availability, appropriateness, and flexibility of one type of service will always have an impact on how other types of service are used. People using long-term care services may have identical treatment and care needs and yet receive services in different settings.

LONG-TERM CARE NEEDS OF AIDS PATIENTS

Increased knowledge about HIV/AIDS, new drugs, earlier intervention, and improved treatment protocols have all had an impact on changing the type and severity of the clinical illnesses that characterize the course of HIV disease. These improvements in treatment mean that people frequently survive episodes of acute illness and sometimes go on to a relatively stable period with few or no symptoms, and others may remain significantly incapacitated. Although stabilized, these people often need prolonged treatment to complete their recommended course of therapy and sometimes need lifelong maintenance therapy once the initial course of treatment is completed. For example, people with *pneumocystis carinii* pneumonia will require medications intravenously until their respiratory systems are controlled and will then take oral medications for the rest of their lives. There are also many chronic disorders that do not reach acute stages for which prolonged treatment is also required.

In all these instances, it is the type and degree of functional incapacity that determines whether there is a need for long-term care services. There is no clearly defined point at which it is appropriate to refer someone with AIDS for long-term care services. The need for services occurs largely as a result of the interrelationship between functional disability, social circumstances, and resource availability. *Functional disability* means that someone has difficulty providing care for themselves, which includes monitoring of the health care condition; medical treatments, such as taking medications regularly and safely; assistance with personal care such as bathing, dressing, and eating; and care to maintain their household, such as shopping, cooking, and light cleaning.

People with AIDS in general may have functional disabilities that result from general weakness, from the effects of particular HIV-related infections, from AIDS neuropsychiatric disorders such as dementia, from depression and isolation, from side effects of drugs used for treatment, or combinations of any of these factors. These functional disabilities may be complicated when the older person with HIV/AIDS has preexisting chronic health care problems.

Long-term care services are intended to respond to problems in functioning by providing rehabilitation, health care monitoring and treatment, and assistance with activities of daily living. Rehabilitation services can assist people in regaining functioning and to help people compensate for functioning that has been lost. In situations in which rehabilitation is not possible, other long-term care services can be put into place.

The kinds of chronic problems that may result in referrals for physical, occupational, or speech therapy include fatigue, shortness of breath, problems in swallowing, visual impairments, contractures, peripheral nervous system (PNS) and central nervous system (CNS) damage, spinal cord dysfunction, stroke, and pain management. People with PNS and CNS damage, for example, show evidence of gait changes, impaired balance, general mobility problems, changes in muscle tone, loss of fine motor coordination, tremors, and general weakness, and sometimes these conditions can be helped by physical therapy, occupational therapy, or both (Galantino & Pizzi, 1991).

When a rehabilitation therapy assessment is done, the patient should be assessed and treated not just from a performance perspective (whether he or she can do the personal, health-related, or household task), but also from the perspectives of the time of day certain tasks are performed, the environment in which they are performed, and the extent to which these tasks are of value and importance in the life of the older person with AIDS. Specific assessments should also be done of strength, range of motion, coordination, muscle tone, sensation, endurance, and cognition. They should also include a determination of the patient's former as well as present routines of daily living in order to assess the physical and psychosocial skills that may require therapeutic intervention for an adapted routine (Galantino & Pizzi, 1991).

Long-term care services may be needed to closely monitor a patient's health condition, sometimes on a daily basis, or at least more frequently than would be feasible through regular visits to the health care provider. For example, some medications used to treat AIDS and related infections can produce severe, life-threatening side effects such as suppression of bone marrow, anemia, and other blood disorders. Some can cause psychiatric symptoms such as insomnia, confusion, hallucinations, mania, and depression, as well as toxicity presenting as delirium (Clark, 1991). Evaluation for these and other symptoms can be performed in the person's home.

The kinds of assistance with personal or household care that may be needed include help with shopping and meal preparation. Adequate nutrition, and sometimes even the physical act of eating, are frequently problems for people ill with AIDS. Help with household or personal care may also be needed when functional disability occurs because of one or more of the neuropsychiatric disorders associated with AIDS: dementia, delirium, depression, and delusions. Cognitive deficits may include memory impairment, mood changes, decreased concentration, slight to severe aphasia, mental slowing, and impaired judgment.

In addition, AIDS patients may experience depression, apathy, anxiety, fear, and social isolation, all of which are common problems for persons facing a life-threatening illness. People with HIV/AIDS and a history of injecting drug use are more likely to have issues of poverty, homelessness, transient life styles, discomfort with structured programs or settings, and general poor health even before AIDS, all of which can have a negative impact on functional ability. Some AIDS patients may need continued substance use treatment. All of these psychosocial issues are intimately related to how someone handles functional disability and life-threatening or terminal illness (or may be disabling factors themselves) and need to be considered when planning and delivering effective long-term care services.

Finally, people with AIDS, especially older adults, have to confront at various times in the progress of their illness decisions about whether to continue with aggressive treatment or to seek more palliative care. Palliative care interventions focus more on quality-of-life issues and relief of symptoms. Not all long-term care services are equally able to provide both aggressive treatment and palliative care.

HOME CARE

Within the range of long-term care services provided to those with AIDS, home care has played by far the most significant role, due to a variety of factors: (a) care at home, or in a homelike atmosphere, is perceived to be preferable to institutional long-term care; (b) the majority of those who have been ill with AIDS have been younger and, to a significant degree, able to draw on the support and assistance of friends, family, and volunteers; and (c) the lack of access for people with AIDS to other formal long-term care programs left a void that home care was uniquely able to fill because the service itself is so flexible and requires almost no capital investment. Home care has also been very successfully combined with other services such as housing, adult day health, hospice, and shelters to meet the needs of all people with AIDS, including older persons.

The range of home care services available has included personal care services, skilled nursing care (including tube feedings, suctioning, and IV therapies), physical and occupational therapies, speech and language pathologists, psychiatric services, and hospice care. Sometimes, the first service that home care programs have to provide is assistance in negotiating the complicated process of applying to entitlement programs, which may be necessary because the person with AIDS no longer has the physical or mental capacity to do so (Clark, 1991; Wyatt, 1990).

What makes home care so flexible is the ease with which different types of service can be initiated or discontinued and hours of service increased or decreased depending on need. Because the condition of AIDS patients can change so rapidly, this flexibility is particularly important.

The Visiting Nurse Service in New York City, which has provided home care services to people with AIDS since very early in the epidemic, stated that their average period of service has increased over time and is now 7 months (Wyatt, 1990). However, included in this average are a number of clients who have stayed much longer, in some cases as long as 2–3 years.

Overall, most AIDS patients receiving home care services have required more coordination time than other patients. The reasons for this include the unpredictability of HIV disease and the sometimes rapid onset of new infections, as well as the fact that people with AIDS are often involved with many other programs—volunteer or otherwise—with whom coordination and collaboration is necessary (Swan, Benjamin, & Brown, 1992; Wyatt, 1990).

The degree to which home care services are available to people with AIDS varies greatly, depending primarily on geography. Large cities are most likely to have specialized AIDS home care programs, even more so since monies have become available through Ryan White federal funding. However, even in areas where there are no specialized programs, home care for people with AIDS is far more common now than it was a few years ago. The question in small towns or rural areas is more likely to be whether there is ready access to providers, hospitals, or nursing facilities with expertise in treating people with HIV/AIDS.

There is also great variability in the amounts and types of service available, depending on both locale and financial resources. Although even 24-hour professional nursing care (by registered nurses) is paid for by Medicaid and is available in some circumstances, it is extremely rare. More typically, home health services are available for a few hours each day, or for a few days a week, with professional nursing visits as needed. Home care agencies offering hospice services often make their services available to people with AIDS. However, rehabilitation or psychiatric services are not always available. In addition, there may be circumstances in which an older person with AIDS has access to Medicare-covered services that younger people with AIDS do not have.

Basically, whether the older person with HIV/AIDS is cared for at home will depend on geography, financial resources (including insurance, Medicaid, or Medicare), the kind and amount of care needed, and the availability of a caregiver for those hours in the day when there is a need for care and home care services are not available.

There are some circumstances when care cannot be safely provided in the home, such as when the person with AIDS has dementia and is unable to direct his or her care and there is no other person who can take significant responsibility for overseeing that care. This situation may occur even more often in an older population with HIV/AIDS whose support system may also be disabled or have died. Safe care can also not be ensured in home care settings without phones when technological interventions are being administered, as undesired reactions to the medications can be quite severe and require emergency treatment; in homes without running water for significant lengths of time; and where there are ongoing criminal activities such as sale of illegal drugs.

Although home care has many advantages, it can also leave the patient very isolated. This is an emerging problem among elderly persons, who are sometimes homebound for years at a time. Not surprisingly, therefore, many of the programs used in conjunction with home care, such as congregate housing settings and adult day health programs, are organized to respond to the social as well as the health care needs of those they serve.

HOUSING

Although there is by no means enough housing available for people with AIDS, estimates are that more than 6,000 beds have been developed by more than 400 programs located around the country (Chen, 1993). These include special rent subsidy programs, assisted access to Section 8 housing, emergency housing, transitional housing, shared rental programs, independent living programs, supportive housing, and residential hospices (Lieberman & Chamberlain, 1993).

Rent subsidy programs provide additional monies to AIDS patients for their rent so that they may remain in their own homes and not run the risk of becoming homeless. Section 8 housing is a U.S. Department of Housing and Urban Development program that allows certain tenants to pay 30% of their income for renting privately owned apartments that meet specified criteria. Emergency housing is often a shelter where many people share a common sleeping and bathroom space. Transitional housing programs are used most often for people who are awaiting permanent placement, and sometimes support services, including home care, are available in these settings. Some programs make apartments available, on a shared basis, to two or more people with AIDS with some support services. Other programs have organized independent living settings, where tenants have their own room and access to cooking and common living areas. There are a number of different models for supportive housing, but the intent is always to make a wide variety of support services available. Residential hospices provide some support services and are usually affiliated with organized health services as well.

Many communities have some but not all of these programs available, whereas many others have none of these services. The issue here, as with other AIDS-specific programs, is that the congregate programs tend to be targeted to younger people. This need not be a barrier, but it is a consideration. Older people may also have access to a wider variety of housing-related programs such as age-restricted housing and senior citizen rent exemptions.

ADULT DAY HEALTH CARE

Day programs were introduced to the United States from England in the 1960s as an alternative to institutionalization. There are basically three day program models: the mental health day treatment model, the adult social day care model, and the adult day health care model. Adult day health care programs most commonly serve frail elderly persons, and basic services include nutrition, medical, and nursing services; rehabilitation; social services; recreation; and transportation (Mason, 1993).

The first adult day program specifically for people with AIDS opened in New York City in 1988, and since then a few other AIDS day programs have opened across the country. Although these programs are not all identical, for many clients the programs function as the primary coordinator of a variety of needed services and are able to make many of them available in one central location. Program components added specifically for people with AIDS include intravenous drugs–nutrition and chemotherapy, aerosolized pentamidine therapy, and blood transfusions (Lieberman & Chamberlain, 1993; Mason, 1993).

These programs can be extremely helpful in sustaining people who otherwise are homeless or live in substandard housing or who live in relative isolation in single-room-occupancy dwellings or their apartments. Frequently, they have insufficient income to eat properly or to purchase medications. Not uncommonly, they have a history of substance use, and many have neurological manifestations of AIDS, including dementia. The opportunity for social interaction and support is an especially critical component of the program (Mason, 1993; Wyatt, 1990).

There are only a few AIDS-specific day programs at present, and it is not known what percentage of the clients using these facilities are over age 50. Although there are instances in which people with AIDS have been admitted to adult day care programs targeted to elderly persons, this is not common.

NURSING HOMES

Because AIDS is complex and unpredictable, more than the standard level of complexity is required of a nursing home that provides care to AIDS patients. It should therefore not be assumed that every long-term care institution is equipped to provide the kind of care that AIDS patients may need. This is extremely important because ignoring this issue could result in a lack of needed care for AIDS patients who are sent to a long-term care facility if it is assumed that all facilities are equally able to respond appropriately and effectively when this is in fact not the case.

Although many facilities resist admitting people with AIDS because of concerns about infection control, about admitting people who have a history of drug use or who are openly gay, and about the reaction of other residents and families, there is now considerable evidence to support the fact that, with proper preparation and education, these issues can be dealt with and should not in themselves be an impediment to admitting people with AIDS. Issues that can, however, be more difficult for a facility to address are the potentially more sophisticated and more intensive care requirements, adequacy of reimbursement, and concerns about how best to respond to the episodic nature of the disease (Wyatt, 1989).

Without question, some AIDS patients do need nursing home care, usually because the resources available to them are not sufficient to meet their needs. This may happen because home care is not available enough hours of the day; because the patients are homeless, have inadequate housing, and therefore cannot have home care; or because they are alone and the onset of dementia has caused them to be unable to direct their own care. However, many, if not most, AIDS patients choose to continue receiving aggressive treatment throughout most of their illness. Even at a point late in the disease process when many overriding functional incapacities may have developed, new episodes of infection can occur. Given the complexity of the disease and the resulting diagnostic and treatment requirements, many nursing homes will find it difficult to meet these needs. AIDS patients will often have not only more complicated, more intensive, and a wider variety of medical and nursing needs, but also more extensive psychosocial requirements (Afzal & Wyatt, 1989; Blustein, Schultz, Knickman, Kator, Richardson, & McBride, 1992; Kator & McBride, 1990).

Essentially, the additional resources needed include strong ties to an acute care facility with AIDS expertise, physician and nursing knowledge and experience with people with AIDS, additional nurse and nurse aide staffing to be made available as needed, and access to drugs needed for AIDS care. Some drugs used in AIDS treatment are new; others are common but very expensive when used with the frequency that AIDS patients tend to need them. An additional consideration is whether the AIDS patients in the facility have a history of substance use. When this is the case, it is frequently necessary to obtain onsite expertise in substance use treatment.

Many nursing homes across the country do have the capacity to deliver good

AIDS care. Some facilities have set aside a group (a floor or a wing) of beds for AIDS patients, and in this way have focused appropriate resources (such as more intensive nursing and physician services) so that services can be developed and concentrated more effectively, thus permitting a more efficient and coordinated approach. Although a few communities have developed AIDS-only nursing homes, it is not necessary to do so to provide appropriate services to people with AIDS.

The issue of adequacy of reimbursement rests to some extent on how many AIDS patients are being cared for in a particular setting. The effect will depend on the overall case mix (and reimbursement system) and on the average demands on the home's resources. Care for one or two AIDS patients may not make that much of a difference, but caring for a number of people with AIDS in one setting is more resource-intensive and more costly than caring for a similarly sized group of more typical patients. Palliative care, however, may not require the same degree of acute care backup and may be easier (and less expensive) for the average home to provide. Unfortunately, palliative care is not always readily available in many nursing homes where it is not uncommon for someone near death to be sent to the hospital. Palliative care is, of course, available in hospice settings, which are discussed in the next sections. In general, however, nursing homes have less experience with responding to the needs of someone in the terminal stage of a difficult and often painful illness. Furthermore, although most hospitals are not reimbursed to provide long-term care services for some patients who are close to death, it may be more appropriate to keep them there rather than transfer them to a nursing home. It is often not possible to predict when death is near with AIDS patients (Nokes, 1994), but when it is possible to do so, it may be more humane not to transfer the person to unfamiliar surroundings, and it may also be a better use of limited resources (Wyatt, 1989).

The fact that the needs of AIDS patients tend to fluctuate greatly can be a problem, not so much when they are sick, but when they are feeling better. In between episodes of infection or other illness, patients can be well for long periods when they may not need any care at all. At such times, institutional life can be very constraining, and arranging to return to the community is sometimes difficult or impossible.

A recent report prepared by the American Health Care Association (1994) from data collected by the Health Care Financing Agency directly from nursing homes across the country has indicated that there are more than 1,700 beds currently available for people with AIDS. Some states had none, or fewer than 10, whereas New York had fully one third of the beds. However, this report noted only those beds considered to be part of special care units, which means that there are probably more beds actually available that are not in special care units. Given the number of people ill with AIDS, this is still a small number. It is difficult to know, however, where the bed shortages actually are, as the need for the beds tends to depend not only on the prevalence of AIDS in a given community but on the variety and amount of other AIDS services. For example, some communities may have small housing programs with 24-hour home care or hospice care available and may therefore not need nursing home beds. However, there are many communities, particularly in small towns or rural areas, where there are no AIDS services at all.

In this context, it may be easier for nursing homes that have not previously provided AIDS care to consider doing so if the person applying is older and would typically be entering a nursing home, regardless of the AIDS diagnosis. However, it would still be important to ascertain whether the facility can provide the appropriate level of service—aggressive treatment or palliative care—and there is always the danger if not the likelihood that being the only AIDS patient in such a facility would be a very isolating experience.

Alternatively, AIDS-specific nursing home programs are generally geared to younger patients, even if they are part of facilities that also serve a traditional nursing home population. As was mentioned earlier, such settings need to be sensitive to the needs of older people that may exist apart from AIDS.

HOSPICE CARE

Hospice services have played an important role in providing long-term care to people with AIDS, but not as central a role as was initially anticipated. This is true primarily because people with AIDS have generally been reluctant to accept hospice services, preferring instead to continue aggressive treatment for as long as possible. In addition, although many hospices have provided a great deal of AIDS care, and in some cases have been the first long-term care programs in their community to do so, not all hospice programs have participated as fully. Finally, most hospice services emphasize care at home, but some people with AIDS live in inadequate housing or have no home at all or no one to help with their care on a daily basis (Beresford, 1993; Wyatt, 1990).

Providers of hospice care for people with AIDS have generally fallen into one of the following categories: (a) Medicare-funded, home-care-based programs, with inpatient care available; (b) non-Medicare-funded, home-care-based programs, also with inpatient care available; (c) highly structured, medically oriented inpatient programs; and (d) congregate housing settings that often but not always are tied into organized health services.

Hospice programs provide palliative care to people who are within a few months of dying (in Medicare-funded programs, a physician must certify that death is anticipated within 6 months). Most programs provide this care to people in their own homes (Medicare-funded programs assume that patients will only require about 20% of the time on an inpatient unit, if that, and will be at home the rest of the time).

Providing hospice care for AIDS patients, however, has generally been more complicated than providing such care for more traditional hospice patients. Aggressive treatment is not part of hospice care, and yet even after entering a hospice, there are some AIDS patients who, although they know they are dying, wish to continue with experimental drugs. Some treatments and drugs that can alleviate symptoms for AIDS patients are also not normally considered "palliative" in a hospice setting, including some IV treatments. Also, it is not always possible to predict when someone with AIDS is within 6 months of dying.

Furthermore, AIDS patients have usually required much more time as inpatients than other hospice patients, often because their housing situations could not support hospice care. This, along with added drug costs, has generally made hospice care for AIDS patients more expensive than care for other hospice patients.

Older people may sometimes be more able than younger people to accept the fact that they are dying and may therefore be more willing to consider hospice care. However, the ability of individual hospices to address the issues regarding which drugs and treatments are considered palliative for AIDS patients, the frequent need by AIDS patients for additional inpatient care, and the resulting increased costs will vary from program to program, largely depending on funding sources as well as on the overall commitment of the program.

SUMMARY

In reviewing the long-term care issues of people with AIDS, three issues stand out. First, it is especially interesting to note that AIDS long-term care services have developed in ways that often cross the usual long-term care service delivery lines. The frequent mixing of housing, home care, and hospice care is the most obvious example. This clearly arose from the need to compensate for the fragmentation found generally in the long-term care continuum, and the development of models that address the integration of health and social needs has been a significant contribution to the field of long-term care. Second, AIDS-specific services have dominated the delivery of long-term care to people with AIDS and have been essential to the process of defining standards for appropriate care. Certainly, consumers tend to prefer AIDS-specific long-term care. However, if long-term care is to become more widely available, greater integration will be necessary. Finally, the very fact that older people with AIDS have to think in terms of two separate service delivery systems is itself an indication of how fragmented chronic health and social services have become. When greater integration of services occurs, then older persons and society as a whole will greatly benefit.

REFERENCES

Afzal, N., & Wyatt, A. (1989). Long term care of AIDS patients. *Quality Review Bulletin, 15*(1), 20–25.

American Health Care Association. (1994). *Total special care beds—1994* [Health Care Finance Agency's online survey: Certification and reporting data]. Washington, DC: Author.

Benjamin, A. E. (1989). Perspectives on a continuum of care for HIV illnesses. *Medical Care Review, 46*(4), 411–437.

Beresford, L. (1993). *The hospice handbook.* Boston: Little, Brown.

Blustein, J., Schultz, B., Knickman, J., Kator, M., Richardson, H., & McBride, L. (1992). AIDS and long-term care: The use of services in an institutional setting. *AIDS & Public Policy Journal, 7*, 32–41.

Brant, L. (1991). Psychosocial concerns of HIV-infected individuals. *Journal of Home Health Care Practice, 3*(2), 52–58.

Chen, T. (Ed.). (1993). *Conference report.* Seattle: AIDS Housing of Washington.

Clark, J. (1991). HIV nursing management in the home health care setting. *Journal of Home Health Care Practice, 3*(2), 1–9.

Galantino, M. L., & Pizzi, M. (1991). Occupational and physical therapy for persons with HIV disease and their caregivers. *Journal of Home Health Care Practice, 3*(3), 46–55.

Kane, R. A., & Kane, R. L. (1987). *Long-term care: Principles, programs, and policies.* New York: Springer.

Kator, M., & McBride, L. C. (1990). Developing a long term care facility program for AIDS patients. *PRIDE Institute Journal of Long Term Home Health Care, 9*(1), 15–19.

Lieberman, B., & Chamberlain, D. P. (1993). *Breaking new ground.* Seattle: AIDS Housing of Washington.

Linsk, N., Cich, P., & Cianfrani, L. (1993). The AIDS epidemic: Challenges for nursing homes. *Journal of Gerontological Nursing, 19*(1), 11–22.

Mason, L. (1993). *Making connections: Adult day health care for people with AIDS* (Report for the United Hospital Fund of New York).

Nokes, K. (1994). Living with AIDS. In B. Backer, N. Hannon, & N. Russell (Eds.), *Death and dying: Understanding and care* (pp. 183–200). Albany, NY: Delmar.

Robert Wood Johnson Foundation. (1994). *Making connections: AIDS and communities.* Princeton, NJ: Author.

Swan, J. H., Benjamin, A. E., & Brown, A. (1992). Skilled nursing facility care for persons with AIDS: Comparison with other patients. *American Journal of Public Health, 82*(3), 453–455.

Wyatt, A. (1989). The consumer's perspective: Matching patient needs with service capacity. In D. L. Infeld & R. M. F. Southby (Eds.), *AIDS and long term care* (pp. 79–89). Owings Mills, MD: National Health.

Wyatt, A. (1990). AIDS and the long term care continuum. *PRIDE Institute Journal of Long Term Home Health Care, 9*(1), 6–13.

Chapter 8

Legal and Ethical Issues

Kathleen Carver
A. Widney Brown

Older persons with HIV may face a variety of legal problems that younger persons with HIV do not have. In exploring the context of these legal problems, it is important to identify the special needs and issues of this population. Two major groups are affected by this trend: older gay men and older members of ethnic minorities. Their experiences with the legal system before seroconversion are crucial factors in determining how they deal with legal issues arising out of their HIV infection.

As discussed in chapter 6, gay men make up the largest group of older persons with HIV. These are gay men who came of age and lived in a United States in which survival as a gay man required living dual lives—a public one as a heterosexual (sometimes married and with children and sometimes the perennial "eligible" bachelor) and a fiercely private one as a "closeted" gay man. To be found out was to risk losing family, job, and prestige. Now, as more and more of these men face HIV, they are caught between being "outed" by their HIV infection and dwindling resources that may force them to seek assistance from the very institutions that have been perceived as threatening as they walked the tightrope of their sexuality and the safety of being closeted.

Therefore, any discussion of legal issues for older people infected with HIV must acknowledge that the very institutions that this population has learned to avoid may be the institutions best suited to helping them make the choices they are confronted with. Even as these institutions become less homophobic, the prevalence of ageism and residual homophobia make the navigation of crucial legal institutions perilous. In practical terms, this means that some older gay men will choose not to be tested for HIV for fear of inappropriate disclosure; they will not issue advance directives; they will be denied the right to participate in studies for experimental treatments; they will be subjected to abuse by people charged with caring for them as they become incapacitated; and they will become increasingly isolated as their support system is devastated by AIDS. In short, these men will face the risk of shedding their dearly maintained privacy in the hopes of receiving fair, compassionate treatment from the very institutions that a mere 2 decades earlier would have destroyed them.

The second largest group of older persons with HIV are members of racial and ethnic minorities, particularly African American and Latino persons. These groups also face particular obstacles when trying to address their legal needs. Like gay men, racial and ethnic minorities have a long history of mistreatment at the hands of the legal system. Some older persons are immigrants who may or may not have legal documents to stay in the United States. Those who are undocumented may avoid seeking any services, including legal services, because of their fear of being deported or punished.

Even for persons legally residing in the United States, language barriers and lack of familiarity with various institutions may deter them from seeking the help they need. Legal processes are universally laborious, intimidating, and confusing. Although most court systems provide interpreters for people who are not fluent in English, the interpreters are not necessarily trained or willing to identify and assist clients in understanding all the permutations of the legal process. Older persons may be dependent on younger family members who are fluent in English to assist them in negotiating the legal system. However, this puts people with HIV in the position of revealing their status to their families and may raise conflicts of interests. For example, the person charged by the family with interpreting for the client may benefit from a specific outcome to the legal proceeding that is contrary to the wishes and best interests of the client.

Furthermore, the inescapable nexus between poverty and race in the United States presents another obstacle for older persons with HIV. These clients are less likely to receive adequate legal representation or health care and may be more vulnerable to being exploited by unscrupulous people, including those pedaling "miracle cures."

Complicating the lives of all older people with HIV is the general lack of respect and attention given to them in the United States. These groups are dealing with their life-threatening illness in a society that patronizes and marginalizes them. One of the most important functions that a health or social service provider can perform is that of making referrals to agencies sensitive to the myriad issues that clients confront on the basis of their sexual orientation, ethnicity, class, and HIV status, as well as age.

In this chapter, HIV and age-related issues concerning discrimination protections, advance directives, guardianships, wills, euthanasia, access to experimental treatments, access to long-term care, and elder abuse are explored. (See

Appendix B for resources for legal services and a list of state statutes that provide civil rights protections on the basis of sexual orientation.)

DISCRIMINATION

For older persons with HIV, the struggle to survive is undermined by the pervasive and pernicious discrimination based on age as well as on HIV status. The following provides a basic review of antidiscrimination protections that the authors hope will assist health care providers in talking with clients about their rights and in making appropriate referrals for clients who experience discrimination in one or more areas.

Although discrimination claims can sometimes be brought outside of court without legal assistance, individuals who think they may have a discrimination claim should be encouraged to consult with an attorney. Among other things, an attorney can assist in moving a case along through administrative agencies charged with enforcement, where a backlog of cases may result in a case being dropped or delayed. In larger cities, legal assistance for HIV-infected persons can often be obtained at a low cost, if not free of charge, through AIDS service organizations. In communities with fewer resources, individuals should be encouraged to consult with any existing civil rights organizations for referrals.

Although certain states provide for strong antidiscrimination protections, the strongest and broadest federal protection is provided by the Americans with Disabilities Act (ADA). Passed by Congress in 1990, the ADA protects people with disabilities from discrimination in private settings, including employment, education, and business settings. The ADA also prohibits state and local governments from discriminating against persons with disabilities in government programs. HIV disease is considered a disability and falls under the purview of the ADA (American Civil Liberties Union, 1993).

The ADA's protections extend broadly to all aspects of HIV disease, including asymptomatic infection. The ADA protects against discrimination that can be linked to a mistaken belief that an individual is infected or has been exposed to HIV through association as a friend, lover, family member, buddy, or caretaker of an HIV-infected person. The ADA also protects people with addictions from discrimination once they are in recovery, although active substance abusers are not protected (ADA, 1990).

Employment Protections

The Americans with Disabilities Act. Although employers are naturally concerned about an HIV-infected employee's ability to adequately perform his or her job, many HIV-infected employees, including people who are aging with HIV, are perfectly capable of performing the essential requirements of their positions. The employment protections afforded by the ADA should be kept in mind for aging people with HIV who wish to remain employed or who are seeking employment. Employment protections are particularly important as most people's sense of self-worth is intimately connected to their ability to contribute to society, such as through work. It is important for older persons with HIV to remain employed for as long as they wish because it provides the worker with independence and reduces direct costs associated with loss of health insurance and disability benefits.

As of July 1994, any business that employs more than 15 people is covered by the ADA, and some state and local laws may cover smaller employers. Under the ADA, a covered employer cannot refuse to hire a person simply because he or she has or is believed to have HIV disease. The following additional points should be kept in mind regarding employment protections under the ADA (American Civil Liberties Union, 1993):

1. An employer cannot fire or refuse to promote someone based on their HIV status.
2. The fact that an HIV-infected person might become too sick to work in the future cannot legally serve as an excuse for refusing to hire or for firing the person now.
3. To fall under the protections of the ADA, an HIV-infected person must be otherwise qualified to perform the substantial responsibilities of the job, despite illness. Although the disabled person's inability to perform a peripheral function is not grounds for refusing to hire, he or she must be well enough to get to work on a regular basis and to perform the job adequately.
4. The employer must make "reasonable accommodations" for persons with disabilities. The employer has the responsibility to make changes in a job that will help the person perform the job adequately. However, the employee has the responsibility to initiate such accommodation by requesting it.
5. Depending on the size of the employer and the nature of the workplace and the job, reasonable accommodation could include establishing flexible work schedules and allowing time off for medical treatment. Other accommodations an employee with HIV may need include the following: job reassignments to positions with reduced physical exertion and stress, reduced hours, more breaks, use of labor-saving equipment, and work-at-home arrangements.
6. The employer is required by law to make accommodations that are "rea-

sonable," that is, accommodations that will not impose "undue hardship" on the employer. This determination of undue hardship is never a purely mathematical exercise. A large employer may be required to spend a substantial amount of money to accommodate an employee while a small employer may be able to argue that even a fairly minor expenditure creates an undue hardship. Thus, any determination will be made on a case by case basis.

7. For people who are already employed, the results of an HIV test cannot be used as grounds for firing a person. For job applicants, an employer may require an HIV test if it is required of all applicants for the same or similar job positions. However, an HIV test can only be required after an actual job offer has been extended, and the offer generally cannot be withdrawn on the basis of the results of the HIV test unless the employer can demonstrate that there is a valid, medically founded reason why a person's HIV-positive status would interfere with the employee's ability to perform an essential function of the job. All employers and agents of the employer who may learn of an employee's HIV status should keep the information confidential pursuant to laws regarding the confidentiality of medical records.

8. The remedy for violation of the employment portion of the ADA is that a written complaint must be filed with the Equal Employment Opportunity Commission (EEOC) within 180 days of the alleged incident, and before filing a lawsuit. For information or the address of a local EEOC office, call 1-800-669-4000 or write to 1801 L St., NW, Washington, DC 20507.

When an ADA claim is substantiated, an HIV-infected employee who has been fired or treated unfairly has a right to reinstatement with back pay or to receive compensation for discriminatory treatment. Discrimination is less difficult to prove when an action to terminate or a pattern of harassment begins immediately or soon after an employee's HIV status becomes known at his or her place of employment. If an employer tries to mask discriminatory intent behind pretextual excuses, an HIV-infected employee can counter such attacks by demonstrating a history of receiving positive work reviews, promotions, and/or merit raises. In each case, the treatment of an employee should be comparable to that of any other similarly situated employee. For example, if all of the employees in a department routinely arrive 15 minutes late, firing an HIV-infected employee for being chronically late may be evidence of discriminatory intent.

Employment protections under the Age Discrimination in Employment Act. For aging persons with HIV, the Age Discrimination in Employment Act

(ADEA) may provide an alternative mechanism for combating employment discrimination. The ADEA was enacted by Congress in 1967 to protect older employees from victimization because of stereotypes about age and the ability of older employees to perform a job. The ADEA mandates equal treatment of rather than a preference for older workers and generally prohibits job discrimination against workers between the ages of 40 and 70.

The ADEA applies to employers, labor organizations, employment agencies, and state and political subdivisions. Although most claims allege discrimination between an individual in a protected age group and an individual under age 40, the statute also prohibits discrimination on the basis of age between two individuals within the protected age group. The ADEA provides not only for back-pay awards but also for liquidated damages in the event of willful employment discrimination. Administration and enforcement of the ADEA is vested in the EEOC.

Family and Medical Leave Act. The Family and Medical Leave Act (FMLA), which took effect on August 5, 1993, guarantees eligible employees the right to take unpaid leave from a job for family or medical reasons. The FMLA applies to private employers who, within a 75-mile radius of the employer's work site, employ 50 or more persons for each working day for each of 20 or more calendar work weeks in the current or preceding calendar year.

To be eligible for FMLA's protection, the employee must have been employed for at least 12 months and for at least 1,250 hours during the prior 12-month period. Eligible employees must be provided with an unpaid leave of up to 12 weeks in any 12-month period for a variety of health-related reasons, including birth or adoption of a son or daughter; care of a son, daughter, spouse, or parent of the employee with a serious health condition; or because of a serious health condition of the employee that prevents the employee from performing the functions of his or her position. The employer can require certification by a health care provider. Providing pay during the leave of absence is at the employer's discretion. Eligible employees are generally entitled to be restored to their old job or an equivalent position with equivalent pay and benefits. Employment benefits that may have accrued to the employee before the date of leave cannot be lost or taken from the employee.

The Employee Retirement Income Security Act. The Employee Retirement Income Security Act (ERISA) prohibits an employer from taking action against an employee that is designed to deprive him or her of benefits under ERISA-protected plans. Health insurance is clearly an ERISA benefit. However, difficulties can arise when a health plan decides not to cover an illness, specifically

AIDS, at a stated point in time. The question of whether those with HIV can be denied health insurance coverage is currently being litigated in the courts.

The Civil Rights Act of 1964. The Civil Rights Act of 1964 prohibits discrimination in employment on the basis of sex, religion, national origin, race, or color. Acts or practices that disproportionately affect persons in these protected categories, as well as intentional acts of discrimination directed at these protected groups, are prohibited. The statute, however, does not protect persons from discrimination on the basis of their sexual orientation, nor does it provide protection for undocumented workers.

Although many have argued that a constitutional basis exists for prohibiting discrimination on the basis of sexual orientation, the U.S. Supreme Court has declined to recognize one. The Supreme Court upheld the right of states to enforce antisodomy statutes, saying there was no privacy right to engage in homosexual relations, even between consenting adults and even in the privacy of one's own home (*Bowers v. Hardwick*, 1986). The dissent vehemently argued that the right of an individual to conduct intimate relations in the privacy of his or her own home is at the heart of the Constitutional protection of privacy. However, given the current composition of the Supreme Court, it is unlikely that *Bowers v. Hardwick* will be overturned in the near future.

Public Accommodation Protection

The ADA offers a variety of non-employment-related antidiscrimination protections. The public accommodation provisions of the ADA cover essentially every type of business and service provider, regardless of size and regardless of whether they receive government funds.

Under the public accommodations portion of the ADA, people with disabilities are protected against discrimination by physicians, dentists, pharmacists, and all other health care providers; hotels, restaurants, movie theaters, convention centers, and health spas; bakeries, clothing stores, and any business that provides commercial services; museums, parks, and schools; and homeless shelters, adoption agencies, and any place that provides social services. The provision also applies to all federal, state, and local government entities. Only religious organizations and private clubs are exempt from the public accommodations provisions. The provision can be enforced by filing a lawsuit in court or, when discrimination is by state or local government, by filing a complaint with the Department of Justice. For more information, call 1-202-514-0301 or write to the Department of Justice, Office on the Americans with Disabilities Act, Civil Rights Division, U.S. Department of Justice, P.O. Box 66118, Washington, DC 20035-6118.

The Fair Housing Act

Discrimination in the sale or rental of private housing is prohibited under the Fair Housing Act (Fair Housing Act as Amended, 1988). A landlord may not refuse to rent an apartment to and may not evict a tenant because of his or her perceived or actual HIV status. The antidiscrimination provisions of the Fair Housing Act are enforced by filing a lawsuit in court or by filing a complaint with the Department of Housing and Urban Development (HUD). HUD complaints must be filed within 1 year of an incident. For the location of a HUD office in your area, call 1-800-669-9777 or write to HUD at 451 Seventh St., SW, Washington, DC 20410.

ELDER ABUSE

Probably no abuse problem is more hidden, undocumented, or ignored in this society than the issue of elder abuse. What few studies exist have hypothesized that 5%, or 1.5 million older people are abused each year in the United States. The abuse takes many forms. Physical abuse appears to be the most prevalent, with financial and psychological abuse following. When the older person is infected with HIV, the justification for the abuse is reinforced by a society that all too often blames the victim.

A 1992 survey conducted and published by the National Association of People with AIDS cited as its most startling finding the result that nearly one third of all respondents had been specifically targeted for violence because of their HIV status. Combining these figures with the statistics on elder abuse, service providers are working with a population that is extremely vulnerable to violence and abuse.

A person being abused may fear that turning to the criminal justice system will result in disclosure of HIV infection and retaliation at the hands of the abuser. It is imperative that social service providers, legal service providers, and health care service providers be trained to recognize symptoms of elder abuse. Once a case of elder abuse has been identified, the abuser should be identified and options to protect the abused person should be explored. If the abuser is a family member, the victim may have the option of going to family court. If the abuser is not a traditionally recognized family member, the survivor may have no choice but to press charges through the criminal court system. This can be a draining and traumatic experience. The survivor should be apprised of any programs to assist persons who are older, disabled, or both. Many district attorneys' offices throughout the country have liaisons to specific groups.

Where the abuse is such that it does not rise to the level of a crime (e.g., harassment), other options should be explored, including mediation and concili-ation. If the abuser has a professional relationship with the victim, the victim should be assisted in filing appropriate complaints. For example, if the abuse is taking place in a hospital or a long-term-care facility, complaints should be filed with the administrator or patient representative and the state's department of health.

The fears of older people with HIV and their reluctance to turn to institutions that may be homophobic, racist, or ageist further complicate this problem. For example, anecdotal evidence has suggested that some older gay men may choose to provide lodging for a younger man in the hopes that this person will take care of them as they become ill. All too often, this unofficial arrangement turns exploitative and abusive. However, the choice to deal with problems of physical incapacity through arrangements that cannot be monitored reflects the fear that many older gay men have of being institutionalized and stigmatized. These noninstitutional arrangements, rather than providing the hoped-for escape, can become traps for the person who becomes isolated from other resources and support.

Older persons may turn to family members for long-term nursing care, espe-cially in cultures in which the tradition of care is firmly rooted in the extended family. However, the physical, emotional, and financial needs of the patient–family member may become overwhelming for the family, especially as younger members of the family become increasingly assimilated in a culture in which older members are not valued and are routinely relegated to institutions.

The care that the patient chooses may be inadequate and may lead to abuse and neglect. Although institutions such as nursing homes, home health care programs, hospitals, and hospices may be homophobic and racist, in most states such institutions and agencies are closely regulated, and complaints may be filed with an oversight agency if internal complaint procedures fail to remedy the problem.

Another form of abuse that older persons with HIV may be subjected to includes the negligent or willful failure to diagnose HIV infection. As seen in the preceding chapter, it may be negligent in that the health care provider may not consider the possibility that an older person could be HIV-positive. As report after report emphasizes that AIDS is becoming a leading cause of death among younger members of society, the destruction wreaked by AIDS among older members of society is overshadowed. This manifests itself in the failure of HIV service providers to teach prevention, including safer sex protocols, to older persons, particularly postmenopausal women; the failure to routinely screen older persons for high-risk behavior; and the failure to diagnose an HIV infec-tion. Older persons with HIV may be excluded from participating in experimental treatment programs. Researchers justify these exclusions by arguing that it is too cumbersome for the persons conducting the experiment to control for the different medications that an older subject may be taking. Vigorous advocacy on a client's behalf may eradicate some of these barriers to experimental treatments.

Older persons with HIV who are institutionalized may be segregated from the other patients in the institution. Such segregation has been found illegal, as there exists no medically indicated basis for segregating persons with HIV. However, many institutions have bowed to the pressure of employees and clients whose irrational fear of being infected causes them to demand quarantine and segregation. Because the fear is irrational, such policies are vulnerable to legal challenges.

PLANNING FOR INCAPACITY

Older clients, especially those infected with HIV, will eventually have to plan for the possibility of incapacity that renders them unable to look after their financial affairs and physical needs. Before clients reach the first stages of incapacity, it is important to counsel them to make appropriate arrangements for the future. Although many clients will be resistant to discussing the impact of mental incompetency and physical incapacity, it is vital that clients be made aware of the importance of planning for the future. Furthermore, once the plans are made, the clients often feel a sense of relief that they have gotten their houses in order.

Each state offers a variety of options. The following are discussed in this section: power of attorney, guardianship–conservators, and guardianship of dependent children. Each jurisdiction has its own terms and statutes controlling these roles. Clients should be advised to ask their legal service providers to explain the options available in their state.

A durable power of attorney gives power to an agent designated by the client before incapacity. Arranging for a person to have power of attorney avoids the necessity for the court to appoint a guardian, conservator, or both. A springing durable power is available in some states and allows the agent of the client to handle the client's affairs when the client becomes incapacitated enough to require the agent's intervention. The most sophisticated springing powers allow for the power to be terminated if the client regains his or her capacity.

Generally, guardians are court-appointed persons responsible for looking after the client's welfare. Conservators are court-appointed persons responsible for looking after the client's property and assets. It is important that when an older person is diagnosed with AIDS that the natural memory loss associated with aging not be misdiagnosed as AIDS-related dementia, resulting in prematurely taking control from the client. Thus, no legal actions should be undertaken without first ensuring that a thorough physical and psychological assessment has been conducted by a qualified and neutral person.

Power of Attorney

Designating an agent to hold the client's power of attorney is the least restrictive form of control. The client chooses the agent, defines the parameters of the power conferred, and can even specify under what conditions the power shall take effect. When a client is mentally strong but unable to conduct certain transactions because of the physical requirements (e.g., meetings, negotiations, court appearances), the appointment of an agent to have power of attorney with respect to a specific project is an attractive choice. If the power of attorney is to continue in the event that the client becomes mentally incapacitated, it becomes a durable power of attorney. All 50 states and the District of Columbia recognize a durable power of attorney. To be valid, the creation of a durable power of attorney must be in writing and must explicitly state that the power is to continue after the principal becomes disabled or incapacitated. When drafting a power of attorney, it is advisable to list specific powers and authorities to ensure that should the principal become incapacitated, she or he will not be left in limbo as the courts explore whether the agent has the power to make specific decisions.

A client may give the agent power to conduct any necessary business but restrict when the power is conferred. This creates a springing durable power that allows the client to define the situation in which she or he relinquishes control. In some states, should the client recover from the incapacity, the power can literally "spring back" to the client.

An agent designated as having the power of attorney is required by law to act in the client's best interest. However, the appointment of the agent does not require court action. The courts will only get involved if the ethicality of the agent is challenged.

Guardians–Conservators

Sometimes a client will become mentally incompetent and physically incapacitated before an agent can be appointed. In this situation, a person other than the client can ask that the court appoint a guardian–conservator. The first issue to confront in this situation is whether the client is actually sufficiently incapacitated to require a court to appoint a guardian–conservator. An accurate diagnosis of the degree of mental incapacity is critical at this point. An AIDS diagnosis is not sufficient to create a nonrebuttable presumption of AIDS-related dementia. Likewise, age alone is not sufficient to create a presumption of incapacity. An assessment should be made by a competent authority who takes into consideration natural and commonplace memory loss among older people.

Guardianships–conservatorships are theoretically subject to rigorous due process considerations. However, these due process considerations are ineffective if the person subject to the proceedings is not aware of his or her right to be heard. Whenever possible, information regarding a person's right to challenge guardianship–conservatorship proceedings should be disseminated to the persons vulnerable to the abuse. Unfortunately, many state laws are procedurally inadequate, substantively archaic, and demeaning. Widespread corruption and abuse abound. These laws are subject to constitutional challenges, but the very nature of the proceeding makes challenge unlikely unless persons vulnerable to the applications of these laws are aware of the dangers and willing to challenge them.

Where guardianship–conservatorship laws have been challenged and subsequently modified, a clear picture of due process requirements has emerged. For a guardianship–conservatorship proceeding to meet these requirements, all interested parties and especially the person subject to the proceedings must receive actual notice in plain language. When the subject's first language is not English, the person has the right to have a translator explain the proceeding. If the person subject to the proceeding wishes to participate, the court must make a reasonable effort to hold the hearing in such a manner that makes it accessible, including holding a hearing at the person's bedside if the subject is capable of participation. The person subject to the proceeding has a limited right of counsel. This right to counsel attaches when (a) the subject requests it, (b) the subject protests the proceedings, (c) the petition for guardianship–conservatorship is made on an expedited or emergency basis, (d) there exists a conflict of interest with the court-appointed evaluator, and (e) the court determines that the subject should have access to counsel.

The guiding legal criteria of whether to appoint a guardian or conservator depends on the presence of the following factors: a functional lack of capacity, the lack of capacity affects decision-making ability, and the subject's decision is likely to cause him or her to suffer harm.

If these criteria are met, an appointment should be ordered by the court. A provider can be instrumental in recognizing when a person subject to a guardianship–conservatorship proceeding is being unfairly subjected to this action and can explain that the subject does have due process protections and encourage that person to insist that those protections be provided.

Finally, any person subject to guardianship or conservatorship proceedings should be clearly informed of the legal effects of such an appointment. In the eyes of the law, the person loses his or her legal capacity. This means she or he may not enter into contracts, initiate a law suit, marry, or change residency and may be prohibited from making the simplest choices about his or her life. The impact of the loss of legal capacity should not be underestimated.

Guardianship of Dependent Children

As HIV sometimes infects multiple generations of one family, an older family member who is infected with HIV may be the primary caretaker or guardian of young children or teens. In a court proceeding to establish the legal guardianship of a minor, the criteria to be used is the best interest of the child. If the parent's choice of guardian is subject to challenge, the proposed guardian's HIV status may be raised in court. HIV infection alone cannot be the legal basis for denial of custody. Likewise, a grandparent's or parent's visitation rights may be challenged. Courts have held that HIV infection per se does not provide a basis for denying or reducing visitation rights of a noncustodial parent or grandparent.

LAST WILLS AND TESTAMENTS

Drafting a will is a sensible act for anyone old enough to own property and have obligations. Yet most people, regardless how practical they consider themselves to be, avoid the act of drafting a will. Older persons infected with HIV are no different, yet, particularly for gay men or lesbians who may have not traditionally recognized relationships in which they have combined their resources to acquire joint assets, the importance of a will cannot be understated.

Intestate Statutes

Each state has intestate laws that apply specific rules of distributions of assets in the absence of a will. None of these intestate laws recognize gay or lesbian relationships. Therefore, a surviving partner can be financially devastated. This can mean losing a shared home, money in shared bank accounts, and other shared assets. To battle this disposition of assets is not only difficult in light of intestate statutes but also requires that the surviving partner reveal and prove the relationship, a concept that may be antithetical to the surviving partner's very concept of survival.

Validity of a Will

Even when a person drafts a will, it may be subject to challenge. Therefore, if a person is suffering from AIDS, particularly AIDS-related dementia, it is important that when a will is being drafted and signed that there be a medically astute witness to the will who can testify that the testator was competent at the time of the reading and signing of the will.

The laws governing estates and wills vary from state to state. Most states recognize that the competency of the person at the moment of signing the will is critical. Therefore, even if a testator has suffered from memory loss or even dementia, she or he is not automatically incapable of drafting and signing a valid will, as long as she or he is competent at the moment of verifying the will. Some states allow for the witnesses to sign affidavits attesting to the competency of the testator and the validity of the will at the time of the signing. These affidavits are then accepted by the court as valid if the will is challenged. If the testator is concerned that a witness may become unavailable for any reason, arranging for these affidavits is a good idea.

The other challenge facing a survivor is the issue of undue influence. The testimony of a social or health care provider can be invaluable in undercutting the argument that a gay man or lesbian who protects his or her surviving partner from financial ruin is being unduly influenced by that surviving partner.

For a client who is married, it is important to check the appropriate jurisdiction's statutory overrides. For example, so long as a heterosexual couple is married, New York law requires that the surviving spouse be entitled to a statutory share of the estate regardless of the provisions of the will, although the surviving spouse can choose not to elect to receive that statutory share. This underscores the need to write a will with the advice of a lawyer.

Finally, various states have statutes that restrict the ability of the executor and witnesses to receive bequests designated in the testamentary instrument. Therefore, a lawyer should be consulted regarding the choosing of an executor.

PLANNING FOR HEALTH CARE

Advance Directives: Health Care Proxies and Durable Power of Attorney for Health Care

In addition to planning for distribution of property and for guardianship, aging persons with HIV illness should be encouraged to plan for their future health care goals. Indeed, the Patient Self-Determination Act (42 U.S.C.A. § 1395cc(a)(1)-(f)(1)(A), 1990), a federal statute, requires health care providers to distribute written information to all adult patients as to their rights under state law to make decisions about their medical care. The Patient Self-Determination Act applies to hospitals, skilled nursing facilities, home health agencies, hospice programs, and health maintenance organizations that receive Medicaid or Medicare funding. Under the act, patients must be given information on the policies of the provider on implementing their rights under state law. The provider is required to ask whether the patient has executed an advance directive and to document the individual's response. Providers are prohibited from discriminating against a patient on the basis of whether an advance directive has been executed. Finally, providers are charged with the responsibility of ensuring compliance with their state's law on advance directives and to provide staff education on the subject of advance directives (Furrow, Johnson, Jost, & Schwartz, 1991).

Although living will (discussed later in this chapter) legislation has been passed by a majority of states, the preferred planning mechanism where it is available is use of a health care proxy or durable power of attorney for health care. Living wills or medical directives are more useful when used in conjunction with a health care proxy than when used alone. The process of designating a health care agent is usually a simple one. Most states require that a proxy be a written instrument, signed by the person making it and signed by witnesses. Generally, the patient's attending physician is prohibited from serving as the agent. A proxy is easily revoked by orally revoking it or by creating a subsequent proxy.

When a patient designates a health care agent, the proxy is activated only on the patient's incapacity. The person chosen as a health care agent can stand in the incapacitated patient's shoes and make decisions for the patient in consultation with health care providers. Health care proxy statutes usually require that an agent honor the patient's wishes and values to the extent they are known, but a health care agent can usually interpret the patient's wishes as medical circumstances change and make decisions the patient could not have anticipated. These features of health care proxies make them more dynamic and flexible when compared with living wills (Schlesinger & Scheiner, 1991).

A health care proxy is often created to protect a patient's wish to forego life-sustaining treatment, but a proxy can serve other important personal goals as well. For example, designation of an agent can help avoid conflict and tension within a family about who should decide about treatment. For those who have no family members available or who want someone other than a family member to make decisions, the health care proxy provides an important mechanism for consent to treatment. Although family members are explicitly authorized and/or allowed by custom and practice to consent to treatment for an incapacitated adult, individuals outside the family generally have no such authority unless they obtain judicial approval under the appropriate guardianship law. Individuals do not have to provide "clear and convincing" evidence of their treatment wishes if they appoint a health care agent.

Living Wills

A living will is a document by which individuals may express their desires as to the giving or withholding of life-sustaining medical treatment (Schlesinger & Scheiner, 1991). Living wills have been faulted for being either too specific or not specific enough, depending on the circumstances in which they are being applied. Because they are static instruments, living wills sometimes create more problems than they solve. Nonetheless, they remain an important option for people who do not want to delegate authority for health care decisions or who do not have anyone to appoint as a health care agent. The use of a living will as an advance medical directive can augment the proxy as a source of information to support an agent's decisions. This is especially relevant in a state like New York where agents are not authorized to make decisions about withholding food or fluids in cases when they are unaware of the client's specific wishes regarding these.

DEVELOPING AREAS
OF HEALTH CARE LAW AND ETHICS

Two law and policy issues currently being debated reflect divergent attitudes of people suffering from terminal illness. At one extreme, the *futility debate* has arisen around situations in which patients and families may want all possible measures taken, without regard to cost or efficacy. At the other extreme, the issues of physician-assisted suicide and euthanasia arise when patients and families want treatment stopped and also want active assistance with dying.

Futility Debate

Most people would probably agree with the proposition that given limited resources, futile treatments should not be offered. However, there is no agreement as to what constitutes a futile treatment or who has the right to make such a determination. Judgments about futility are less objective than often presumed (Solomon, 1992). A treatment may be deemed futile when a physician judges that a particular patient's life is not worth saving. The decision that certain treatments are not worth pursuing may best be seen as involving a conflict of values rather than as a question of futility (Truog, Brett, & Frader, 1992). For example, although a physician may consider futile a treatment that could keep someone alive in an intensive care unit for a couple of days or weeks, the patient may value those few days or weeks of life highly if he or she is afforded an opportunity to put his or her affairs in order or to see loved ones before dying.

To the extent that value judgments play a role in defining futility, there is valid concern that underprivileged and stigmatized groups may receive less treatment than other groups thought to be of higher social standing. The futility debate crystallized around concerns about rising and seemingly uncontrollable health care costs, advances in technology, and issues of professional autonomy. Older people with HIV living in this era of cost containment may need advocacy around issues of access to intensive care, high-tech treatments, and experimental treatments. Older persons with HIV may be particularly at risk of having their treatment preferences deemed futile by health care providers who are inevitably influenced by society's devaluation of older persons.

Ideally, guidelines for determining futility would be developed not by individual practitioners, but through a process of empirical community agreement. This could serve as a check against subjectivity. However, it has been suggested that in a pluralistic society such as ours, agreement on futility may never be reached.

Physician-Assisted Suicide

Although physician-assisted suicide may be a natural extension of the withholding of treatment for terminal conditions, others believe that it is different because it actively accelerates the dying process. There is a legitimate concern that physician-assisted suicide will be disproportionately used by people who are receiving already inadequate health care or who are generally subordinated in society.

The American Bar Association, the American Nurses Association, and the American Medical Association oppose legalization of physician-assisted suicide, and the laws in many states prohibit people from assisting in suicide. However, physicians compassionately assisting a suicide are generally not vigorously prosecuted, and one state (Oregon) has recently legalized physician-assisted suicide.

The Oregon statute (the Death with Dignity Act) provides the following protections:

- A patient who would be assisted with suicide must be at least 18 years old, be mentally competent, and must be certified by two physicians as having fewer than 6 months to live.

- The patient must request a doctor's assistance in suicide three times, the last time in writing, with the statement signed and dated by the patient in the presence of two witnesses. At least one witness must be a nonrelative with no interest in the estate and cannot be an employee of the hospital or nursing home where the patient is being treated.
- The doctor must wait at least 15 days after the initial request, and at least 2 days after the final written request, before writing the prescription for lethal drugs.
- The patient must get the drug and take it. The law specifically proscribes lethal injection, mercy killing, or active euthanasia.

A doctor who follows these guidelines cannot be prosecuted or disciplined by professional organizations for doing so. A doctor can also refuse the patient's request for a lethal prescription. Killing by lethal injection, mercy killing, and active euthanasia are all explicitly prohibited (Colburn, 1994).

Those who oppose legalization of physician-assisted suicide point out that a request for help in suicide might mask a desperate plea for help by a distraught patient in physical or emotional pain. Physician-assisted suicide may provide a convenient way to get rid of poor or disabled persons, and once physician-assisted suicide is legalized, many fear a "slippery slope" toward euthanasia. Virtually every guideline established by the Dutch to regulate euthanasia has been modified or violated with impunity, so that euthanasia is no longer practiced only for the terminally ill but also for the chronically ill, not only for physical illness but also for psychological distress, and not only voluntarily but also involuntarily (called *termination of the patient without explicit request*; Hendin, 1994).

People who seek assisted suicide generally want to avoid unnecessary suffering and maximize their choices and sense of control in the face of death; however, many argue that these outcomes can be achieved in a more desirable fashion, such as by referral to hospice care. Hospice care makes the relief of suffering the primary objective, allowing use of treatments to alleviate suffering even when a person's life may be inadvertently shortened. Hospice programs are designed to give individuals as much choice and control as possible. For some, physician-assisted death would only become a legitimate option in those infrequent circumstances in which patients are suffering intolerably in spite of excellent hospice care (Quill, 1994).

People with HIV illness frequently consider suicide. When HIV illness is compounded by the problems and stigma associated with aging, suicide may look like an even more attractive option. However, from a policy point of view, it must be kept in mind that physician-assisted suicide is no longer rational when chosen out of the self-hatred or devaluation that follows social oppression.

SUMMARY

Laws have been made to protect the rights of all individuals; this includes older adults with HIV/AIDS. Discrimination against older persons with HIV/AIDS in employment, public accommodations, and housing is illegal, as is elder abuse. Older individuals who plan for incapacity by making legal, financial, and health care arrangements will be in a better position to have their wishes and interests followed. This is especially true in the case of evolving ethics regarding physician-assisted suicide. By working with clients to put these mechanisms into place, helping professionals can ensure that their clients will get the level of care that they want and deserve.

REFERENCES

Age Discrimination in Employment Act 29 U.S.C. §§ 621-634 (1967 & Supp. 1982).

American Civil Liberties Union. (1993). *The Americans with Disabilities Act: What it means for people living with HIV disease.* New York: ACLU AIDS Project.

Americans With Disabilities Act of 1990, 42 U.S.C. § 12101 *et seq.*

Bowers v. Hardwick, 478 U.S. 186, 106 S. Ct. 2841 (1986).

Colburn, D. (1994, November 15). Assisted suicide bill passes in Oregon. Law puts state at center of ethical debate. *The Washington Post,* p. 209.

Employee Retirement Income Security Act, 29 U.S.C. § 510 (1974).

Fair Housing Act as Amended, 42 U.S.C. 3601-3619 (1988).

Furrow, B., Johnson, S., Jost, T., & Schwartz, R. (1991). *Bioethics: Health care law and ethics.* St. Paul, MN: West.

Hendin, H. (1994, December 16). Scared to death of dying. *New York Times.*

National Association of People with AIDS. (1992). *HIV in America: A profile of the challenges facing Americans living with HIV.* Washington, DC: National Association of People with AIDS.

New York State Bar Association. (1995). *AIDS and the workplace.* Albany, NY: New York State Bar Association Special Committee on AIDS and the Law.

Pincus, L. (1993). The Americans With Disabilities Act: Employers' new responsibilities to HIV positive employees. *Hofstra Law Review Association, 21,* 561–600.

Quill, T. E. (1994). Risk taking by physicians in legally gray areas. *Albany Law Review, 57,* 693–708.

Schlesinger, S. J., & Scheiner, B. J. (1991). Planning for the elderly or incapacitated client. In *Tax law and estate planning course handbook.* New York: Practicing Law Institute.

Solomon, M. (1992). Letter to the editor. *New England Journal of Medicine, 327,* 1239.

Truog, R.D., Brett, A. S., and Frader, J. (1992). Sounding board: The problem with futility. *New England Journal of Medicine, 326,* 1560.

Chapter 9

Caregiving Issues

Joan Levine-Perkell

HIV/AIDS is not the exclusive province of youth, but researchers, social scientists, government, and the media have colluded to create this myth by directing the focus of their research and policy efforts almost entirely toward the 40-and-under population. The place of older persons in the AIDS epidemic as recipients, providers, or cosharers of care can no longer be overlooked (Ory & Zablotsky, 1989).

This chapter focuses on caregiving issues surrounding older Americans in the era of HIV/AIDS. Specifically, it explores the special challenges experienced by caregivers of aged persons with HIV/AIDS, elderly parents as caregivers to their children with HIV/AIDS, and grandparents raising grandchildren orphaned by the HIV/AIDS epidemic.

ELDERLY PERSONS INFECTED WITH HIV/AIDS

Typically, AIDS and aging share multiple physical, psychological, and social dimensions. The dynamics of fear, stereotyping, rejection, and stigma are common to AIDS and growing older. Thus, the older person infected or affected by HIV/AIDS experiences a twofold impact of negative social response (O'Neil, 1990). Yet, 14 years into the epidemic, the nation is just beginning to address the issue of older Americans and AIDS.

The physical and emotional devastation of HIV/AIDS in elderly persons produces extraordinary challenges to caregivers and to the health care system. Families of origin and families of choice assume heavy responsibilities for the care of these individuals. Raveis and Siegel (1990) found that even in a relatively healthy sample of persons with AIDS (PWAs), informal and family caregivers provided approximately two thirds of the total assistance required for instrumental activities, transportation, administrative functions, and home medical care (Brown & Cope-Powell, 1991).

Spouses and significant others are often the main source of care for the older PWA. Partners' own advanced ages and concomitant health problems render this group particularly susceptible to serious physical and mental health problems as a consequence of their caregiving. These elderly caregivers are subject to stress associated with performing household tasks, personal care of the patient, increased financial burden, and limited social and leisure activities. Research has demonstrated that family caregivers of elderly or ill persons suffer loss of self (possibly because of the deterioration of an intimate marital relationship or transformation of the "couple identity"; Skaff & Pearlin, 1992), depression (Rankin, Haut, and Keeforer, 1992), mental exhaustion (Livingston, 1985), and burden (Zarit, Topp, & Zarit, 1986).

The literature (Lovejoy, 1988; Maj, 1991) on caregivers of PWAs also emphasizes the added burden, often starting immediately with diagnosis. The first response of the infected person's partner to the diagnosis of HIV infection or AIDS is frequently shock, a narrowing of attention, apathy, and sometimes physical symptoms such as heart palpitations and paresthesias that may require treatment. This reaction can be intensified as the partner encounters unfamiliar medical routines or diagnostic procedures when accompanying the infected person to the health care provider. The sense of shock is often followed by an urgent need on the part of the caregiver to obtain information about the disease, what to expect in relation to the progressive nature of HIV/AIDS, guidelines on sexual behavior, and instruction on domestic hygiene, how the virus is transmitted, and how to support the loved one. After this initial period, anger is often the dominant feeling. It may stem from the perception of lost dreams and aspirations and from the anticipated decline in the quality of life for the infected person and the family (Maj, 1991).

Many times PWAs ask their partners and spouses not to disclose that they have HIV/AIDS. In this way, the caregiver is deprived of the support that may have been derived through interaction with others. This "conspiracy of silence" causes the caregiver to have increased feelings of frustration, stress, and isolation and at times an overwhelming sense of hopelessness. As the disease progresses, caregivers experience additional stress associated with the social stigma of the disease, a decreasing social network as friends and family shy away, anticipatory loss of the relationship with the person for whom they are caring, the strain caused by the heightened awareness of their own vulnerability to the disease, and the many changes in the patient's health status. The family is often, although not always, confronted with news of the infected family member's previously unknown homosexuality, drug use, infidelity, promiscuousness, or prostitution at the same time as that of the diagnosis of a devastating illness (Maj, 1991). In the late stages of the disease, care of the PWA requires enormous amounts of energy. In some cases, caregivers may become totally absorbed in their partner's needs, disregarding their own physical appearance, health, emotional needs, and other relationships. This tremendous involvement may be followed, when the partner finally dies, by the remaining partner's loss of the will to live (Maj, 1991).

In male same-sex couples, the issue of identification of the caregiving partner with the infected partner frequently arises (Pearlin, Semple, & Turner, 1989). The less ill partner may see the infected partner as how he fears he will become in the future and may even foresee a situation in which no one will be left to give him the same care he is now providing. The gay male partner may want to share memories and grief with their deceased lover's family, but family members may want no further contact. This ostracism after death leaves the bereaved partner with a legacy of infection surrounded by a hostile family of origin. To alleviate spiritual discomfort and give meaning to death from AIDS, the gay community has developed rituals that allow public expression of feelings. These rituals create a transitional event, emphasize the continuity of life, and are emblematic of the struggle between the need to hold on and the need to let go (Walker, 1991). In place of traditional religious rites, gay people have created memorial services in which participants let loose balloons to celebrate the release of the soul, have candlelight processions, and have made the AIDS quilt, which joins together the lives of untold numbers of deceased PWAs. Each square of the AIDS quilt is dedicated to the memory of a beloved person. Walker (1991) notes, "In an age that has lost touch with the importance of ritual, the rediscovery of its value in recovering from loss seems critical" (p. 254).

Stall and Catania (1994) noted that the scientific literature regarding risks for HIV has been predominantly concerned with the risk-taking characteristics of the young. Irrespective of whether studies have included injecting drug users, heterosexual persons with multiple partners, gay and bisexual men, or ethnic minority populations, those over the age of 50 are only rarely accorded a separate description or subgroup analysis. This wrongly implies that risk for HIV infection is negligible among older adults.

Care of elderly PWAs as described by Stall, Catania, and Pollack (1989) encompasses care by the medical system, public agencies, families, and social networks as well as self-care. It is often necessary for the caregivers to coordinate the efforts of the various components of the care network in order to create a treatment plan for the patient that takes into account the PWA's ongoing social, emotional, medical, financial, physical, and spiritual needs. This can be overwhelming to caregivers as they try to educate themselves as to the service solutions for the patient's acute and chronic needs, including the coordination of adequate and appropriate housing, home care services, equipment provisions, transportation, and money management. A case manager is needed to assist them in facilitating service integration and delivery.

It is becoming increasingly apparent that HIV infection does not spare people past the age of 50 years. As such, it is appropriate to begin addressing the psychological problems of older caregivers of HIV-infected Americans. The limited available empirical and anecdotal reports have suggested that the impact is very dramatic.

ELDERLY PARENTS OF PERSONS WITH AIDS

The number of AIDS cases reported by the Centers for Disease Control and Prevention (CDC) has been the most widely used measure of the AIDS epidemic in the United States (Des Jarlais, Wenston, Friedman, et al., 1988). AIDS surveillance data are used to monitor trends, assess the future impact of the epidemic, detect new patterns of disease, facilitate the development and evaluation of prevention measures for HIV infection, and guide policy decisions related to the allocation of resources (Rosenblum, Buehler, Morgan, et al., 1992). The greatest number of older adults who are affected by the HIV/AIDS epidemic are the parents of those who are infected, who are symptomatic, or who have died (Riley, Ory, & Zablotsky, 1989). Parents of PWAs reside in every region of the country; they span several generations and have a variety of religions, political affiliations, and cultural heritages. Parents vary greatly in the level of financial, emotional, and physical support that they offer their adult children with HIV/AIDS (O'Neil, 1990). One third of PWAs are dependent on older parents for financial, emotional, and physical support (Allers, 1990). These older caregivers are also confronting their own diminishing capacities (Riley, 1989). In addition, they are often living on fixed incomes (Ory & Zablotsky, 1989) and have limited knowledge of the disease and ways to negotiate the social service system (O'Neil, 1990). In addition, Skeen, Walters, and Robinson (1988) reported that many parents experience the double trauma of learning about their child's homosexuality or substance use at the same time that they learn of his or her HIV/AIDS diagnosis. Carl (1986) referred to this as the *double death syndrome.* Parents must deal with the loss of a "normal" child at the same time that they must deal with that child's illness and impending death as a result of AIDS. Sometimes families of choice and families of origin collide, and there are no socially established behavioral patterns to guide them (Cleveland, Walters, Skeen, & Robinson, 1988).

Several reports have shown that family systems of PWAs are often disrupted by the stigma of AIDS (Christ & Wiender, 1994; Lloyd, 1989; Maj, 1991). Fear of contagion disrupts family gatherings, and families become increasingly isolated. Eventually, the patient's inexorable physical and mental decline leads to demoralization and despair on the part of the caregivers, as well as overt psychiatric symptoms of anxiety and depression. Parents also become angry because of the child's alternate lifestyle, wonder whether other family members knew about it, and may blame the infected child for becoming ill or feel guilty that they failed as parents.

If parents decide to provide care for the infected child, the routines of their daily life are unavoidably compromised, and the stress increases as the adult child becomes sicker. Relationships between the primary caregiver and the rest of the family may become conflicted (Maj, 1991). Issues related to HIV/AIDS may also be shrouded in secrecy and not discussed within the family or with friends or formal caregivers. This silence adds more stress and impairs the ability of family members and friends to comfort and understand each other's issues. In families with a history of multiple losses, the anticipation of a new loss may create tension between the patient and the caregiver that may build to the point of rejection.

Caregivers may also be afraid of becoming infected with HIV or tuberculosis (TB) as a result of their caregiving activities. Transmission of HIV has been reported in homes in which health care was provided ("HIV transmission in household settings," 1994b). A 75-year-old woman cared for her son during the period before his death from AIDS. She provided bathing, feeding, and mouth care; changed diapers; and repositioned his urinary catheter. Although she was instructed to wear gloves when she handled his body secretions, she reported that she did not use them every time. The CDC believes that she became infected with HIV as a result of her caregiving activities ("Guidelines for preventing the transmission of Mycobacterium tuberculosis in health-care facilities," 1994a). Gloves and other barriers must be used every time anyone handles body secretions of PWAs, and hands should be washed with soap and water after the gloves are removed. Appendix C is a handout developed by the U. S. Environmental Protection Agency and should be reviewed with every caregiver.

Because TB is transmitted through the air, the transmission of mycobacterium TB is a recognized risk to caregivers ("HIV transmission in household settings," 1994b). Clients with confirmed or suspected TB should be instructed to cover their mouths and noses with a tissue when they cough or sneeze. Caregivers should be evaluated periodically with skin tests (purified protein derivative) for TB infection as recommended by the CDC ("HIV transmission in household settings," 1994b). Good ventilation will assist in decreasing the TB exposure of people who are living or visiting the home of the person with TB and HIV/AIDS.

An atmosphere of mourning is created as parents attempt to cope with the impending death of their adult child. Studies have shown (Sanders, 1989; Shanfield, Benjamin, & Swan, 1984; Shanfield & Swan, 1984) that the death of a child produces the highest intensity of bereavement, with the death of an adult child being the most traumatic (Gorer, 1965). The resulting grief is extremely prolonged, due to the older parent's social isolation, the parent's own sense of physical and mental decline, and the loss of instrumental support in that the adult child typically is seen as the person who would have assisted the elderly parent as he or she became more dependant. The loss of adult children is perceived as an "out-of-time loss" as parents are "supposed" to predecease their children. In his work with parents who had lost a child, Sanders (1989) described them as giving the appearance of individuals who had just suffered a physical blow that left them with no strength or will. This can be especially devastating to older adults, and may result in a loss of interest in living, thereby accelerating their own deaths.

Doka (1989) has described how the stigma of AIDS creates disenfranchised grief, wherein the usual coping mechanism are disrupted because friends and family deny the disease and the world is seen as hostile and incapable of understanding. Because of this stigma, some survivors fear they will be rejected and judged harshly if the cause of death becomes known. Persons may attribute the death to cancer or some cause other than AIDS. Such deception in the long run takes its emotional toll in fear of discovery, anger that a cover-up seems necessary, and possible guilt over what they have done (Worden, 1991). In addition, many parents blame themselves for their child's alternate lifestyle and behavior. Caregiver stress and stigmatized grief may be reduced in supportive bereavement groups in which parents who have shared similar experiences can ventilate feelings and receive emotional support (Worden, 1991).

Compounding the loss of their adult children, older people are often faced with raising their children's children. Therefore, at a time in life when they should be retiring, they find themselves raising a new generation, their grandchildren. The next section of this chapter examines this issue in detail.

GRANDPARENTING ISSUES

AIDS cases among women were reported almost from the beginning of the epidemic. However, because of the overwhelming impact on gay men, especially White gay men, and the government's and media's almost single-minded focus on this population in the early years, AIDS as a threat to women and children was underestimated (Levine, 1993).

Nearly one half of the women diagnosed with AIDS have been injecting drug users (IDUs), with one fourth of all women with AIDS infected through heterosexual sex with an IDU (CDC, 1993; Michaels & Levine, 1992). In 1992, the number of women infected through heterosexual contact exceeded the number infected through injecting drug use (CDC, 1993). Furthermore, these women are often their families' primary caregivers. When they die, they leave children of all ages (Michaels & Levine, 1992). More than 80% of these children are offspring of African American and Hispanic women (Michaels & Levine, 1992). Because the rate of HIV transmission from mother to child is approximately 25%, it can be estimated that at least one quarter of those children who were delivered while their mothers were infected were also infected with HIV.

Therefore, AIDS has created a cohort of new orphans (Davidson, 1993). The Orphan Project Report (Levine & Stein, 1994) was the first nationwide analysis of surviving children of PWAs and their potential service providers in this era of the epidemic. Levine et al. estimated that by the year 2000, in New York City alone there will be 30,000 children aged birth to 17 years who will have lost their mothers to AIDS. The majority of these children and young adults will not be HIV-infected, will come from poor communities of color (Michaels & Levine, 1992), will be at high risk for a wide range of behavioral and psychological problems (Levine & Stein, 1994), and will require a multitude of services. This tragic legacy of AIDS orphans and the burdens of their new caregivers is a challenge worthy of the best efforts of the public and private sectors.

AIDS has also distorted the typical generational division within families. Grandparents usually remain free of parenting responsibilities in relation to grandchildren. However, because of the AIDS epidemic there is a growing number of grandparents nationwide for whom middle age and late life has become a time of "unplanned parenthood" (Minkler & Roe, 1993). In 1991 the U.S. Bureau of the Census estimated that 3.2 million children under the age of 18 live with their grandparents: 12% of all African American children, 5.8% of all Hispanic children, and 3.6% of all White children. These figures represent a 44% increase in the past decade, a 24% increase in Black children, and a 40% increase in Hispanic children, with White children showing the largest increase, 54% (Jendrek, 1994). One third of these cases are in "skipped-generation families" in which neither biological parent is present and the grandparents have become the surrogate parents (Minkler & Roe, 1993). These numbers are staggering, as they do not represent the entire picture of grandparent caregiving, which may be three or four times worse (Burton, 1992), particularly in inner city areas hardest hit by the AIDS epidemic (Minkler & Roe, 1993). There are uncounted orphans in senior housing facilities that do not permit children and in private homes and apartments where grandparents chose not to fight for legal custody of their grandchildren. The stigma of AIDS keeps these caregivers underground.

Caregiving Stress

Caregiving stress related to a variety of other situations has received considerable attention in geriatric literature (Kelley 1993). Caregiving for one's grandchildren because of the current AIDS epidemic is a new and unique experience (Minkler & Roe, 1993) and has only recently attracted the attention of social scientists. Consequently, there has been relatively little systematic study of the scope and nature of the issues involved (Burton, 1992). The children and their grandparents need more voices.

Michaels and Levine (1992) noted that "The death of a emotionally significant adult is one of the most traumatic experiences that any child can suffer. When the death is accompanied by stigma and isolation and followed by insecurity and instability as it is with AIDS, the potential for trouble both immediately and in the future is magnified. The children can not wait for the normally slow policy process to take account of their complex individualized needs" (p. 3458).

Financial Implications

The media have described the grandparent caregivers in human interest stories as "silent saviors" and "the second line of defense." Limited reports have suggested that grandparents are beset with numerous problems related to the care of this special population of children (Burton, 1992). Recent changes in social and economic conditions challenge the capacity of family networks to provide support for the grandparent who is caring for a minor child (Minkler, Roe, & Price, 1992), yet they get less than one third of the monetary allowance available to foster families (Levine & Stein, 1994). Family caregiving is often unseen and undervalued. In a society predicated on family ethics and stressing duty to care, it is assumed that families will take care of their own. Grandparents are penalized financially for their biological relationship to the children in their care and are denied the support and adequate aid that would assist them in fulfilling a difficult and demanding role (Minkler & Roe, 1993). Funds for disability-related programs are terminated after the HIV-infected parent's death. This loss of AIDS-related assistance may significantly impair the new guardian's ability to care for the surviving children. The problem is especially significant if the guardian has a small, low-rent, or subsidized apartment and cannot afford to move to a different space (Levine & Stein, 1994). Levine and Stein charted the loss of real income to a newly constructed family after AIDS-related subsidies are withdrawn on the death of the parent with AIDS. They estimated that for a parent with AIDS who has two children, the total monthly benefit is $1,932. This is in contrast to the total monthly benefit of $775 for a newly constructed family with two children when the guardian is not on public assistance.

Minkler and Roe (1993) concluded that the decision to care has financial consequences that may be profound, especially in female-headed households. This decision to care is often made in an environment in which Black single females age 65 and older already constitute the poorest group in American society (Grambs, 1989). Many grandparent caregivers have to give up their full-time jobs and incur heavy debts. They are suddenly unable to afford anything but basic necessities, and in some cases not even that (Minkler & Roe, 1993). Minkler and Roe described that, when contrasted with the more substantial financial benefits and other services available to nonbiological foster care parents, the support received by nonrelative caregivers was cause for high levels of anger and resentment.

According to Creighton (1991), the national average for Aid to Families with Dependent Children (AFDC) support was $109 per child per month for grandparents who are caregivers as compared with $371 per child per month for foster parents. In response to legal challenges, California, New York, Maryland, New Jersey, and Illinois have relaxed their licensing requirements to allow grandparents and other kin caregivers to receive payments on par with those of unrelated foster parents (Norris, 1991). Kinship care is becoming the preferred option in order to keep children within their own families. In New York City alone, the children in kinship foster care rose from 45 in 1986 to 23,600 in 1991 ("Sorting out the legalities," 1993). In other states, however, the agencies responsible for foster care payments may refuse financial assistance for children placed with relatives unless the grandparents meet all the same requirements as unrelated persons (Chalfie, 1994)

Legal Status

The many impediments faced by grandparent caregivers can vary on the basis of the legal status of their arrangement, especially if it was not determined before the parents' death from AIDS. Some grandparents seek legally recognized relationships with their grandchildren. Once recognized by law, these grandparent caregivers gain legal and physical custody of the children as well as the right to make decisions for the children regarding their upbringing and the responsibility for the children's daily care (Jendrek, 1994). There are several types of legal relationships—adoption, permanent custody, temporary custody (guardianship), and certification as a foster parent—that qualifies the caregiver for certain state benefits but infers no transfer of custody or parental right. Securing legal custody can be difficult, time consuming, and expensive ("Sorting out the legalities," 1993; see chapter 8).

Grandparent caregivers may informally assume all the daily responsibilities for caring and making decisions about the children, but the arrangement can be challenged. Because there is no official recognition of this living arrangement, these grandparents encounter policy-related problems such as enrolling grandchildren in school, gaining access to school records, and making decisions regarding the child's medical care (AARP, 1994). Many grandparents find it difficult to obtain health care for grandchildren when they do not have legal custody or guardianship ("Parenting Grandchildren," 1994). Some insurance companies do not allow grandparents to cover a grandchild on their own policy, and grandparents with a grandchild on AFDC have reported that they cannot find a pediatrician or general physician willing to accept the AFDC card (Jendrek, 1994).

Studies by Burton (1992), Minkler et al. (1992), and Jendrek (1993, 1995) have described the needs of grandparent caregivers as follows (Jendrek, 1994):

- respite care
- affordable and dependable child care
- increased support and help from human service providers and professional practitioners
- legal advice concerning the implication for obtaining guardianship versus temporary custody, legal custody, or the adoption of the grandchild
- parenting programs
- economic assistance
- tutorial programs
- health care
- job counseling and referral
- drug addiction seminars
- emotional support from peers
- counseling about alcohol, smoking, depression, and anxiety

RELATIONSHIPS

Caregiving duties can change marital, family, and social relationships, and they can isolate the caregiver from former coworkers and friends. Grandparents in despair over their child's illness and death may feel guilty ("If only I'd been a better parent, this never would have happened"). They can also feel angry, resentful, and depressed over second-time-around parenthood (Minkler et al., 1992). As described by Mrs. L, "I have no time for me—I'm the nurse, the secretary, the cook, the housekeeper—I must manage everything for everyone. There is no one there for me—I feel all alone with this." The needs of the dependent grandchild will be greater if that child is also ill from HIV disease.

Burton (1992) reported that 86% of grandparent caregivers were depressed and anxious most of the time, 61% reported increased smoking, 35% reported increased alcohol consumption, 35% reported increased medical problems, 8% reported strokes, and 5% reported heart attacks that they attributed to their caregiving stress. Formal and informal support groups afford caregivers emotional and instrumental support. Group support can address the heroism of the grandparent's effort to keep families together despite minimal reimbursement, neighborhood violence, and havoc wreaked by an adult child's disease and death (Trupin, 1993). In these groups, participants can express feelings of guilt, rage, grief, and resentment; are able to acknowledge the loneliness and depression they are experiencing as the result of multiple losses; and can vent feelings of anger due to the added responsibilities and turmoil associated with the presence of an person with HIV/AIDS in their household. Group members can also address the shortage of social programs and the stigma and shame of AIDS. They may examine the potential health consequences to caregivers, provide HIV/AIDS education, and gain new perspectives regarding parenting in the 21st century and family histories of grandchildren with prenatal exposure to drugs, alcohol, and HIV; exposure to early neglect and abuse; or all of these. These groups empower participants through sharing mutual concerns.

SPIRITUALITY

Religion and spirituality can also facilitate coping responses to illness, loss, and death by softening the burden of living with uncertainty and shame. Burton (1992) indicated that the majority of grandparents experience "the Lord's blessings" in raising their grandchildren. Through coping with multiple losses, grandparents find avenues of renewal and ways of keeping faith and having hope that things will get better (Johnson-Moore & Phillips, 1994).

SUMMARY

Perhaps the needs of grandparents are best verbalized by a 72-year-old grandfather in Burton's (1992) study who said,

We grandparents who are going through these times are all in this together. We are a resource in our community but we need help. We need help to raise these babies to be good men and women. We need help to survive. Sometimes all we need to hear from someone is that we are not alone . . . that someone appreciates the job we are doing. (p. 750)

REFERENCES

Allers, C. T. (1990). AIDS and the older adult. *The Gerontologist, 30*, 405–407.

Brown, M. A., & Cope-Powell, G. M. (1991). AIDS family caregiving: Transitions through uncertainty. *Nursing Research, 40*(6), 338–345.

Burton, L. (1992). Black grandparents rearing children of drug addicted parents: Stressors, outcomes and social service needs. *The Gerontologist, 32*(6), 744–751.

Carl, D. (1986). AIDS: A preliminary examination of the effects on gay couples and coupling. *Journal of Marital and Family Therapy, 12*, 241–247.

Centers for Disease Control and Prevention. (1993). *HIV/AIDS surveillance report* (2nd quarter ed.). Washington, DC: CDC.

Chalfie, D. (1994). *A closer look at grandparents parenting grandchildren: Going it alone.* Washington, DC: American Association of Retired Persons, Women's Initiative.

Christ, G. H., & Wiener, L. S. (1994). Psychosocial issues in AIDS. In V. T. Devita (Ed.), *AIDS: Etiology, diagnosis and treatment and prevention* (pp. 275–297). Philadelphia: Lippincott.

Cleveland, P. H., Walters, L. H., Skeen, P., & Robinson, B. E. (1988). If your child had AIDS . . . Responses of parents with homosexual children. *Family Relations, 37,* 150–153.

Creighton, L. L. (1991, December 16). Silent saviors. *U.S. News and World Report,* 80–89.

Davidson, C. F. (1993). Dependent children and their families: A historical survey of U.S. policies. In F. H. Jacobs & M. W. Davis (Eds.), *More than kissing babies? Current child and family policy in the U.S.* (pp. 65–91). Westport, CT: Auburn House.

Des Jarlais, D. C., Wenston, J., Friedman, S., Sotheran, J. L., Maslansky, R., Marmor, M., Yancovitz, S., & Beatrice, S. (1992). Implications of the revised surveillance definition: AIDS among NYC drug users. *American Journal of Public Health, 82*(11), 1531–1533.

Doka, J. D. (1989). *Disenfranchised grief.* New York: Lexington.

Gorer, G. (1965). *Death, grief and mourning.* London: Cresset Press.

Grambs, J. D. (1989). *Women over forty: Visions and realities.* New York: Springer.

Guidelines for preventing the transmission of Mycobacterium tuberculosis in health-care facilities—1994. (1994a). *Morbidity and Mortality Weekly Report, 43*(RR-13), 1–132.

HIV transmission in household settings—United States. (1994b). *Morbidity and Mortality Weekly Report, 43*(19), 347, 353–356.

Jendrek, M. P. (1993). Grandparents who parent their grandchildren: Effects on lifestyle. *Journal of Marriage and the Family, 55*, 609–621.

Jendrek, M. P. (1994). Grandparents who parent their grandchildren: Circumstances and decisions. *The Gerontologist, 34*(2), 206–216.

Jendrek, M. P. (1996). Policy concerns of White grandparents who provide regular care to their grandchildren. *Journal of Gerontological Social Work*, in press.

Johnson-Moore, P., & Phillips, L. J. (1994). Black American communities: Coping with death. In B. O. Dane & C. Levine (Eds.), *AIDS and the new orphans: Coping with death* (pp. 101–117). Westport, CT: Auburn House.

Kelley, S. J. (1993). Caregiver stress in grandparents raising grandchildren. *Image Journal of Nursing Scholarship, 25*(4), 331–337.

Levine, C. (Ed.). (1993). *A death in the family: Orphans of the HIV epidemic.* New York: United Hospital Fund.

Levine, C. (1994). The new orphans and grieving on the time of AIDS. In B. O. Dane & C. Levine (Eds.), *AIDS and the new orphans: Coping with death* (pp. 1–11). Westport, CT: Auburn House.

Levine, C., & Stein, G. L. (1994). Orphans of the HIV epidemic: Unmet needs in six U.S. cities. In *The Orphan Project report.* New York: The Orphan Project.

Livingston, M. (1985). Families who care. *British Medical Journal, 291*, 919–920.

Lloyd, G. A. (1989). AIDS and elders: Advocacy, activism and coalitions. *Generations, Fall*, 32.

Lovejoy, N. C. (1988). Family and caregiver responses to HIV infection. In G. Gee & T. A. Mortan (Eds.), *AIDS: Concepts on nursing practice* (pp. 379–401). Baltimore: Williams & Wilkins.

Maj, M. (1991). Psychological problems of families and health workers dealing with people infected with human immunodeficiency virus I. *ACTA Psychiatrica Scandinavica, 83*, 161–168.

Michaels, D., & Levine, C. (1992). Estimates of the number of motherless youth orphaned by AIDS in the United States. *Journal of the American Medical Association, 268*(24), 3456–3461.

Minkler, M., & Roe, K. (1993). Grandmothers as caregivers: Raising children of the crack cocaine epidemic. Newbury Park, CA: Sage.

Minkler, M., Roe, K., & Price, M. (1992). The physical and emotional health of grandmothers raising grandchildren in the crack cocaine epidemic. *The Gerontologist, 32*(6), 751–762.

Norris, M. (1991, August 30). Grandmothers who fill the void carved by drugs. *Washington Post*, pp. A1, A4.

O'Neil, M. (1990). AIDS, HIV and older clients. In B. Generay & R. S. Katz, (Eds.), *Countertransference and older clients.* Newbury Park, CA: Sage

Ory, M.G., & Zablotsky, M. (1989). Notes for the future: Research, prevention, care, public policy. In M. N. Riley, M. G. Ory, & D. Zablotsky (Eds.), *AIDS in an aging society—What we need to know* (pp. 202–216). New York: Springer.

Parenting grandchildren. (1994) *The Brookdale Newsletter from the AARP, 1*(2), 1.

Pearlin, L. I., Semple, S. J., & Turner, H. (1989). The stress of AIDS caregiving: A preliminary overview of the issues. In I. B. Carles, L. Pihman, & M. Lindeman (Eds.), *AIDS: Principles, practice and politics* (pp. 279–289). Washington, DC: Hemisphere.

Rankin, E. D., Haut, M. W., & Keeforer, R. W. (1992). Clinical assessment of family caregivers in dementia. *The Gerontologist, 32*(6), 813–821.

Raveis, V., & Siegel, K. (1990). Impact of caregiving on informal or familiar caregivers.

In *Community based care of persons with AIDS: Developing a research agenda.* (DHHS publication numbers PHS 90-34; 56; pp. 17–28). Washington DC: U.S. Government Printing Office.

Riley, M. W. (1989). AIDS and older people: The overlooked segment of the population. In M. W. Riley, M. G. Ory, & D. Zablotsky (Eds.), *AIDS in an aging society—What we need to know* (pp. 3–26). New York: Springer.

Riley, M. W., Ory, M. G., & Zablotsky, D. (Eds.). (1989). *AIDS in an aging society—What we need to know.* New York: Springer.

Rosenblum, L., Buehler, J. W., Morgan, M. W., Costa, S., Hildalgo, J., Holmes, R., Lieto, L., Shields, A., & Whyte, B. (1988). The completeness of AIDS case reporting: A multisite collaborative surveillance project. *American Journal of Public Health, 82*(11), 1495–1505.

Sanders, C. M. (1989). Comparison of adult bereavement in the death of a spouse, child and parent. *Omega, 10*(4), 303–322.

Shanfield, S. B., & Swan, B. J. (1984). Death of adult children in traffic accidents. *The Journal of Nervous and Mental Disease, 172*(9), 533–538.

Shanfield, S. B., Benjamin, A. H., & Swan, B. J. (1984). Parents' reactions to the death of an adult child from cancer. *Journal of Psychiatry, 141*, 1092–1094.

Skaff, M. M., & Pearlin, L. I. (1992). Caregiving: Role engulfment and the loss of self. *The Gerontologist, 32*(5), 656–664.

Skeen, P., Walters, L., & Robinson, B. (1988). How parents of gays react to their children's homosexuality and to the threat of AIDS. *Journal of Psychosocial Nursing, 26*(12), 7–10.

Sorting out the legalities. (1993). *AARP Bulletin, 34*(9).

Stall, R., & Catania, J. (1994). AIDS risk behaviors among late middle aged and elderly Americans: The National AIDS Behavioral Surveys. *Archives of Internal Medicine, 154*, 57–63.

Stall, R., Catania, J., & Pollack, L. (1989). The social epidemiology of AIDS and HIV infection among older Americans. In M. Riley, M. Ory, & D. Zablotsky (Eds.), *AIDS in an aging society—What we need to know* (pp. 60–76). New York: Springer.

Trupin, S. (1993). Moral support for grandparents who care. *American Journal of Nursing, 93*(4), 52–56.

Walker, G. (1991). *In the midst of winter: Systematic therapy with families, couples and individuals with AIDS infection.* New York: W. W. Norton.

Worden, W. J. (1991). Grieving a loss from AIDS. In *AIDS and the hospice community* (pp. 143–150). Hawthorne Press.

Zarit, S. H., Topp, P. A., & Zarit, J. M. (1986). Subjective burden of husbands and wives as caregivers: A longitudinal study. *The Gerontologist, 26*, 260–286.

Chapter 10

HIV/AIDS and Aging Networks

Daphne Joslin
Marie C. Nazon

This chapter describes why organized networks of professionals in HIV/AIDS and aging have been developed by examining the needs that gave rise to such networks, their organization, and activities. The chapter is designed to encourage and support the development of such networks through which professionals from the HIV/AIDS and aging service arenas can address shared concerns and initiate collaborative activities in the service of older adults infected with and affected by HIV/AIDS. Specifically it addresses the following: Why should the HIV/AIDS and aging service networks consider working with one another in a collaborative undertaking? What can be learned from the history of three HIV/AIDS and aging task forces? What are the challenges and benefits of bringing together professionals from these two service systems? How can such a network be organized?

WHY SHOULD A FORMAL NETWORK OF AIDS AND AGING PROFESSIONALS BE DEVELOPED?

A network of HIV/AIDS and aging professionals can form the basis for a range of activities, including individual case conferencing, staff training and development, client/patient advocacy, systemwide advocacy initiatives to address funding, program development, and reimbursement. The need for such networks is described in the following paragraphs.

First, epidemiological and demographic trends continue to place older adults at the center of the HIV/AIDS epidemic (Stall & Catania, 1994). Given these trends, service providers in both fields will increasingly confront HIV/AIDS as an aging issue. Not only are 10% of diagnosed AIDS cases among persons 50 and older, but as HIV/AIDS has become more of a chronic disease, service providers are seeing the "aging in" of the HIV-positive population. Individuals infected in their 40s will be older adults—in their 50s and 60s—when living with HIV disease.

The lack of sufficient targeted HIV outreach, education, and prevention strategies means that in all likelihood the level of HIV infection among older adults is likely to continue, particularly among poorer mid-life older adults of color and women. As HIV/AIDS has evolved from an acute disease to a chronic one with long-term care needs, older adults and persons with HIV/AIDS (PWAs) have come to share the same service systems, such as residential care facilities (e.g., nursing homes), adult day care, and home care. As this occurs, education of older people, their families, and staff members is necessary to allay fears, dispel myths and anxieties, and ensure dignified and humane care (Kern, 1989).

Older relatives have become surrogate parents to thousands of children orphaned by the epidemic. Persistently high and increasing rates of heterosexual transmission of the HIV virus among women of childbearing age will mean an intensification of this unprecedented trend of absent or incapacitated parents and surrogate parenting by grandmothers and other older relatives.

Over the course of the epidemic, older adults have been and continue to serve as the primary caregivers to PWAs: partners, spouses, children, grandchildren, and friends. Current estimates are that at least one third of all persons living with HIV disease are cared for by an older relative (Allers, 1990).

Second, service providers in both the aging and HIV/AIDS service systems are seeing greater numbers of older individuals who are infected with or affected by HIV/AIDS. Often clients present with service needs that can only be partially met within one service system. Holistic strategies for addressing the needs of older clients infected with and affected by HIV/AIDS require that programs and professionals stretch themselves beyond narrow program boundaries.

One of the many lessons learned from HIV/AIDS work with older adults, as with other areas of health and human services, is that individual needs and experiences transcend rigid boundaries of service systems (Fleishman, Mor, Piette, & Allen, 1992). Too often, health and social service delivery is organized according to bureaucratic procedures, eligibility criteria, and reimbursement formulas rather than in response to the needs of the person. Fragmentation in human service is common, not only in HIV/AIDS and aging, but for other client groups as well. "One-stop" service agencies, where client access to multiple services, benefits, and entitlements can be achieved through a visit to one agency, are an example of a concrete strategy to address such fragmentation. Organized networks of professionals in HIV/AIDS and aging services help to bridge this service fragmentation that often pigeonholes individuals into easy categories of eligibility by helping to develop pathways for client referral and case conferencing. Particularly in large metropolitan areas, the individual professionals from the two service systems may not know one another on a face-to-face or name basis. In smaller cities, although informal connections may be greater, there is still a need for formal articulation through a formalized network to achieve maximum results for clients.

UNDERLYING VALUES, ATTITUDES, AND ASSUMPTIONS

Reducing barriers to service access and utilization must involve attention to underlying values, attitudes, and assumptions in both the HIV/AIDS and the aging service systems. Because HIV/AIDS has struck young adults disproportionately while the impact of the epidemic on older adults has remained relatively invisible, the HIV/AIDS service system has not developed a uniform capacity to address the needs of older adults. Staff training in the HIV/AIDS system has tended to ignore aging-related issues. In addition to ageist assumptions, values, and beliefs that must be addressed in order to ensure effective service delivery to older clients, HIV/AIDS staff training and development must include health issues and aging-related programs and benefits for older adults.

At the same time, the homophobia and AIDS phobia that pervade the larger society extend to aging-related programs as well (Lloyd, 1989). Programs that serve older adults and elderly persons may not be "HIV/AIDS-friendly," thus reinforcing the isolation and marginality that older adults who are HIV-positive, ill with HIV disease, or HIV caregivers often experience. By bringing together staff from these two fields, mutual education and interchange can occur, leading to greater awareness and sensitivity that will improve outreach, case finding, HIV/AIDS education, and counseling of older adults affected and infected by HIV.

HEALTH AND HUMAN SERVICES

In a time of scarce resources for health and human services, HIV/AIDS and aging networks help to address the competition for limited funds fueled by a climate of distinguishing between the "undeserving " and "deserving" groups in need. By bringing together professionals from both the HIV/AIDS and aging networks, the isolation and vulnerability of health and human service programs can be actively addressed as staff develop greater awareness of and appreciation for the client needs of each respective service network. At a time when reactive social policies are threatening to pit one service need and needy population against another—children against elderly persons, HIV/AIDS patients against Alzheimer's disease patients—networks of professionals from two seemingly unrelated areas help educate the public, legislators, and other policymakers regarding the implications of failing to address the scope of health and human needs.

CURRENT HIV/AIDS AND AGING NETWORKS

The history of existing HIV/AIDS and aging networks suggests how such organizations come into being and the activities and goals that define their mission. In particular, such cases help to identify key factors that can support the development of such networks.

New York City HIV/AIDS and Aging Task Force

The largest and oldest network of HIV/AIDS and aging professionals, the New-York-City-based HIV/AIDS and Aging Task Force, was formed in 1991 "to identify common issues between AIDS and aging by . . . bring[ing] professionals from the AIDS and aging networks together to address collectively the impact of the HIV/AIDS epidemic on older adults" (Nazon, 1992, p. 2). Housed in and partially sponsored by the Brookdale Center on Aging of Hunter College, City University of New York, the Task Force has a membership of 35 professionals in the New York City area. Members of the task force have included representatives from the local Area Agency on Aging, the regional office of the Administration on Aging, an academic gerontology education and training center, an academic community health HIV/AIDS education center, a senior center, home care, senior housing staff, aging and HIV/AIDS advocacy groups, geriatric education centers, university schools of nursing and social work; a minority task force on AIDS, an organization dedicated to the social service and advocacy needs of older gay men and lesbians; the municipal corporation that manages New York City public hospitals, clinicians, and older persons with HIV/AIDS. Why did the task force come into being? By 1990, professionals in several service arenas were reporting several concurrent phenomena. First, staff of nursing homes and home care agencies affiliated with Hunter/Brookdale Center on Aging or the Hunter/Mt. Sinai Geriatric Education Center began to identify training needs related to care of older HIV patients and their families. At the same time, senior center staff began reporting to Area Agency on Aging (also the New York City Department for the Aging) that some senior center members, particularly women, were no longer attending center programs because they had to care for grandchildren whose parents had died of AIDS. Home care agencies also began to identify clients who, in the absence of other caregivers, had to assume primary responsibility for either an HIV-ill adult child or a grandchild orphaned by HIV/AIDS. Because of greater sensitivity to aging issues and concerns, the Brookdale Center and other aging-related service agencies more readily identified the needs of older adults with HIV/AIDS and older caregivers. However, the need to actively respond to the convergence of HIV/AIDS and aging issues was recognized by key staff of both public and private HIV/AIDS organizations in the city. Recognizing the importance of this convergence issue for service delivery, staff training, and client advocacy, a full-day training conference was held by the New York City Department for the Aging, which brought together more than 200 participants. Building on the momentum stimulated by the training conference, the Hunter/Brookdale Center on Aging convened a conference the following year that attracted more than 150 participants for a full day of panels and workshops to address policy, advocacy, outreach, and education issues. Among the needs identified by participants at this second conference was that of a task force on aging and HIV/AIDS in the city.

The broad aim of the New York City Task Force is to "generate education, programmatic and policy initiatives in the field of AIDS and aging" (Nazon, 1993, p. 4) in order to address the issues of older adults and their families who are affected by HIV/AIDS. Specifically, the goals of the task force are

- to promote an understanding among the public and professional communities in New York of the social, economic, and political impact of the AIDS crisis on the aging population
- to develop a common agenda to meet the needs of older people and people with HIV/AIDS and to ensure appropriate access to funding and services, both in the community and in the long-term-care setting
- to foster an exchange of skills and biomedical and psychosocial knowledge in the area of AIDS and aging among health care agencies, advocacy groups, provider associations, community organizations, and concerned individuals
- to advocate and enforce the development of appropriate policies, education, training, and research to respond to the special needs of older PWAs and older people involved in caring for those with HIV illness

The intention of the Task Force has not been to duplicate education and training that is already underway but rather to identify the gaps in training needs and develop activities and programs to address these unmet needs. Over the course of its 4-year existence, the New York City Task Force has provided educational seminars on the health care needs of HIV-infected or -ill older persons; psychosocial needs and social service interventions and programs; legal, financial, and entitlements concerns; preparing the agency for addressing the needs of older adults with HIV/AIDS; and caregiving by older persons in the HIV/AIDS epidemic. The Task Force also conducted a Mini-White House Conference on Aging in 1995 to address caregiving issues for older persons caring for someone with HIV/AIDS. In providing training and staff development to professionals in both the HIV/AIDS and aging fields, the Task Force has expanded the number of staff who are both competent within their field and sensitive to the needs of older persons affected by and infected with HIV. It has also conducted outreach and education at senior centers, created a resource bank that includes articles and bibliographic materials, and conducted advocacy through public education and legislative testimony. The Task Force meets bimonthly and continues cross-education among members by inviting guest speakers from the HIV/AIDS fields and conducting sensitivity exercises in both HIV/AIDS and aging. The Task Force has also been instrumental in assisting the media in developing appropriate story lines on the topic of HIV/AIDS and aging. As there is a paucity of information in the media in this area, an accurate portrayal of the issues is important. Presently, the Task Force is developing an educational video on HIV/AIDS and aging in collaboration with the American Association of Retired Persons (AARP).

The four working committees established by the Task Force are as follows. The Education Committee examines issues and conducts activities related to education and training of older adults and professionals, develops curriculum and program models, and reviews available materials on HIV/AIDS and aging. The Health Care Committee investigates issues in long-term-care facilities and policy and advocacy issues related to health care. Committee members have canvassed nursing homes and visited several model HIV/AIDS long-term-care programs. The Communities Committee focuses on how communities are responding to the impact of HIV/AIDS on older adults and the needs of specific communities. A proposed project is a needs assessment of HIV/AIDS and aging services in New York City. Finally, the Linkage Committee links the Task Force with other task forces, organizations, and individuals in order to develop a state, national, and international communications network on HIV/AIDS and aging.

In addition to its yearly calendar of planned activities, through its clearinghouse as well as professional networking functions, the New York City Task Force has been instrumental in helping to stimulate the development of other networks around the country. Those identified as of early 1995 included the

Dade and Monroe Counties, Florida, AIDS and Aging Task Force and the HIV
and Elderly Work Group in Passaic County, New Jersey.

Dade and Monroe Counties, Florida

Responding to an estimated 13% of AIDS cases in Dade County being among
people 50 years and older, the Alliance for Aging, Inc., the Area Agency on
Aging for Dade and Monroe Counties, formed a network of organizations from
the aging and HIV/AIDS fields in 1993. Its stated mission is

> to ensure that the concerns of older people and their families affected by the HIV/
> AIDS epidemic are appropriately addressed in culturally sensitive ways and to
> generate educational, programmatic and policy initiatives in the fields of HIV/
> AIDS and aging. Cultural sensitivity includes languages, belief systems, age, gen-
> der and sexual orientation. (V. Delgado, personal communication, January 27,
> 1995)

The Alliance for Aging was one of the first area agencies on aging in the nation
to participate in HIV/AIDS-related issues that affect elderly persons.

Accomplishments of the Alliance include the creation and distribution of
an AIDS and Aging Fact Sheet that provides information regarding HIV transmission and testing, as well as consumer protection regarding unscrupulous
and fraudulent medical treatment and participation in the International AIDS
WALK Miami '94.

HIV AND THE ELDERLY WORK GROUP

As in New York City where an academically based gerontology center served
as a key agent in bringing together the HIV/AIDS and aging networks, the
Gerontology Program at the William Paterson College (WPC) of New Jersey
helped to stimulate awareness of the impact of HIV/AIDS on older adults that,
in turn, led to the creation of the HIV/AIDS and Elderly Work Group in Passaic
County, New Jersey. In 1993, as a spin-off from participation in the New York
City HIV/AIDS and Aging Task Force, the coordinator of the WPC Gerontology
Program initiated efforts to identify HIV/AIDS-related service needs among older
adults living in the county. Brief presentations concerning HIV/AIDS were given
by the WPC gerontology coordinator to two key networks: the local HIV/AIDS
service network organization, the Coalition on AIDS in Passaic County (CAPCO)
and the Passaic County Office on Aging and local aging services providers who
are funded through the Office on Aging. CAPCO is a not-for-profit organization

consisting of more than 45 member organizations and individual members who provide or use HIV/AIDS-related services. Its mission is to promote HIV health education and prevention, to provide networking and training opportunities for service providers, and to provide policy and program recommendations to governmental agencies to assist in policy planning and decision making affecting HIV-infected persons. The Passaic County Office on Aging is an area agency on aging funded through state and local funds as well as the federal Older Americans Act. Its mission is to coordinate and oversee a broad range of services provided to persons 55 years of age and older in the county, through in-home and congregate services such as senior centers, Meals on Wheels, crime prevention, transportation, information and referral, and case management.

In presentations made to CAPCO and to the Passaic County Office on Aging, service providers (such as senior center directors) and staff from both the aging and HIV/AIDS service areas agreed that HIV/AIDS was an issue affecting a growing number of older clients. Direct service and administrative staff from both networks could readily identify active older clients ill with HIV disease, caring for ill family members, or raising grandchildren. The latter were identified as a special concern affecting growing numbers of clients; HIV/AIDS professionals also projected an increase in these numbers on the basis of their own agency caseloads of HIV-infected women and because New Jersey has the greatest percentage of any state of HIV-infected women. Staff from both networks were interested in learning more about the "other side" (i.e., aging or HIV/AIDS) in order to be better prepared to address current and future clients' needs by sharing information across program boundaries, where possible; to engage in case conferencing; and to identify service gaps and policy issues, particularly in relationship to advocacy for public planning of HIV/AIDS services.

An HIV/AIDS and Elderly Work Group was formed, under the auspices of CAPCO, which serves as the organizational base for the work group by convening meetings, distributing minutes, and giving publicity to the work group to attract new members. CAPCO's newsletter, which has statewide distribution, has helped to raise greater awareness of HIV/AIDS and aging through its publication of three articles on HIV/AIDS and older adults.

The Passaic County HIV/AIDS and the Elderly Work Group disseminates information about HIV/AIDS to local aging and AIDS service providers through workshops and monthly meetings. Using a volunteer acting group that performs a range of health-related skits in north central New Jersey, the work group has also conducted an HIV/AIDS education program for older adults attending nutrition sites (senior centers) in the city of Paterson. These "mini-dramas" present scenarios about the impact of HIV/AIDS on older adults and include a 71-year-old man learning that he is HIV-positive, the female companion of this man telling her best friend this news, and a grandmother talking to her sexually active teenage grandson. Common myths about HIV transmission are dispelled in a format that places HIV/AIDS in the context of older people's lives. The minidramas encourage audience interaction and discussion, as audiences are asked, "What would you do in this situation?" Outreach to other congregate sites, such as senior housing and retirement communities, is being planned. An important goal of the HIV/AIDS education program of the work group is to increase the capacity of older persons to educate younger family members as well as other older adults and to break down the isolation that often confronts older adults who are infected with HIV, ill, or caring for a family member or loved one with HIV disease. Next steps include outreach to aging member organizations, such as AARP, veteran's groups, ladies' auxiliaries, and church groups to address the needs of HIV-related caregivers.

BUILDING A NETWORK: THE CHALLENGES, BENEFITS, AND ORGANIZATIONAL NEEDS

As the three case descriptions suggest, the purpose of an HIV/AIDS and aging network is to enhance the efforts by professional service providers and advocates to address the needs of older adults who are clients of a range of health and human service agencies, including hospitals, clinics, nursing homes, senior centers, home care, and AIDS case management and counseling programs. Such enhancement occurs through training conferences and seminars, newsletters, shared advocacy efforts, case conferences, collaborative needs assessment, and the potential for seeking special funds to support special programming.

Organizing Needs

An HIV/AIDS and aging network exists parallel to and ideally is integrated within the existing service delivery system through membership of both institutions and individuals. How can such a network be created and what are the challenges in this undertaking? What is its organizational form? Development of such a network, particularly in a time of limited staff resources and heavier caseloads with greater service needs, can be daunting, but the experience of a number of HIV/AIDS and aging networks from around the country is that professionals in both fields often bring to their jobs a tremendous sense of commitment and energy.

Beyond individual interest by professionals in the HIV/AIDS and aging fields, what are some of the necessary ingredients to developing such a net-work? The history of some of the cases described earlier is instructive. First, endorsement or sponsorship by service agencies is key to developing such a network in order to permit staff to take time for network-related activities such as meetings, correspondence, and speaking engagements. Gaining official orga-nizational support, especially from top and mid-level administrators, may be an educational process in itself as they may not immediately grasp the relevance of this issue to their agency's mission or clients. Such support helps not only to give staff necessary work time for network-related activities but to legitimize the network itself, which in turn helps to recruit other organizations for mem-bership. Moreover, endorsement if not partial sponsorship of the network will be essential if external private or public funding is to be obtained.

In building a network, it is necessary to ensure a balance between those representing HIV/AIDS-related organizations and those from aging services. It is recommended that the task force be cochaired by individuals representing both the aging and HIV/AIDS networks. Not only does this help to dispel a sense of imbalance in the issues but this shared leadership helps to stimulate and guide training, program development, and policy and advocacy initiatives. In addition, dual leadership also helps to promote the marketing of the organiza-tion to each of the service sectors.

A balance of professionals with experience in direct services to clients, policy, advocacy, and training will help to direct network attention to these different areas of need. It is vital to have professionals who also have experience working with older adults in peer-educated and volunteer capacities (Stuen, 1990). This is important in any aging-related work in order to correct the distortion that can occur in aging services where the focus is on client dependency and passivity. An important strength of an HIV/AIDS and aging network is its mobilization of older adults, both those affected and infected by HIV/AIDS and those who are senior advocates.

Ongoing responsibilities of task force and network coordinators include planning and facilitating task force activities, such as regular meetings, corres-pondence, outreach, grant writing and fund raising, and liaison responsibilities (i.e., representing the work group to other organizations, as well as serving as task force spokespersons to the media and the public). Sponsoring organiza-tions must allow release time to staff for network activities.

Creating formal linkages between AIDS and aging services requires a clear sense of mission, planning agenda, and mechanisms for communication and collaboration. Despite the benefits, there are challenges that can be anticipated in bringing together professionals from the HIV/AIDS and aging service sys-tems.

Challenges

First, there is simply the issue of informed sensitivity to HIV/AIDS on the one hand and aging on the other. HIV/AIDS organizations may feel that older adults are a comparatively small proportion of current caseloads and that younger populations are at greater risk and hence warrant greater attention and staff involvement; that limited resources mitigate against further case finding; and that such individuals can be served by senior organizations. In turn, aging service providers may either be unaware that HIV/AIDS affects older adults or want to avoid dealing with an issue that is associated with stigma. Ageism, homophobia, and AIDS phobia all contribute to barriers among professionals from these service arenas. Few agencies have staff that are initially conversant in the language of both worlds and sensitive to the service and advocacy needs of clients from the other system. It may be easier for aging agencies to talk about grandmothers caring for their grandchildren or mothers caring for their adult children than about older adults and elderly persons who are HIV-positive or have AIDS.

Competition for funds may also detract from agency support and participation. Although the two networks typically receive funding from disparate funding sources, an HIV/AIDS and aging task force is in a unique position to seek funds from both HIV/AIDS- and aging-related funds. Here, certain protocols, such as notifying agency staff when potential competition may arise, are important.

The coordinator's role is a delicate one, helping to guide the task force into productive activities yet striving also for the task force's autonomy. Members must see results to keep motivated and involved. Likewise, if professionals participating in the task force do not receive support and active affirmation of the need to integrate HIV/AIDS and aging work into their agency responsibilities, it is difficult to get continuous participation. Uneven participation in an HIV/AIDS and aging coalition, work group, or task force can be a problem in sustaining ongoing projects or undertaking new ones.

Building a Network: The Benefits

The key to a successful task force or network is face-to-face professional networking and cross-education. Networking will enable staff to gain access to information, referrals, and services in the other service network and thereby enhance the ability of staff to address client needs. Staff from aging agencies who are not familiar with HIV/AIDS will have an opportunity to learn about people with HIV/AIDS and their service needs, and staff from the HIV/AIDS organizations will in turn learn about aging. Moreover, professionals and agencies themselves will receive support from colleagues facing similar challenges.

Technical assistance to agencies will enable them to initiate their own training, outreach, or program development with the support and guidance of others with greater expertise. Providing comprehensive and up-to-date information on HIV/AIDS and aging enables clinicians to maximize continuing education in this area and to integrate their own specialization with new knowledge and perspective. Participation in the organized network of HIV/AIDS and aging professionals also provides the opportunity for good public relations for participating agencies. Network members and sponsoring agencies have an opportunity to showcase their agency at meetings, training sessions, and conferences. Where possible, some participating agencies may be able to share resources such as special staff, facilities, training equipment, and transportation.

Participation in the network may also assist agencies in identifying service gaps and new service models, seeking funding alone or in consort with other programs.

How Can Such a Network Be Organized?

One of the first steps in organizing an HIV/AIDS and aging network or task force is to identify organizations and individuals in the community who are interested in aging and HIV/AIDS issues. Initial meetings should be held to identify salient issues pertaining to service needs, gaps, and availability. Common concerns and areas for mutual professional training, community outreach, staff development, and client and systemwide advocacy help set the stage for attracting potential participants. A lead agency or agencies should be identified that will be responsible for maintaining and guiding the network. If funding is available, a coordinator should be selected. A formal organizational structure should be established and cochairs selected. A mission statement, network goals, and objectives should be determined. Regular meetings during this formative stage will help solidify the network's mission and member participation. Meetings and committees should be open to the public to attract greater lay support and interest. Committee goals should be established, and regular progress reports shared with the entire network. Media contacts should be developed through press releases and interviews. Development of a small, attainable project such as a fact sheet on HIV/AIDS and aging or a training conference will help to publicize the organization and also keep the momentum and participation of members and supporting agencies. Participation of community leaders should be sought. Where possible, cosponsorship of programs on HIV/AIDS or aging will also help to market the organization and attract new members.

SUMMARY

In a climate of scarce resources for health and social service needs, as well as persistent homophobia, ageism, and political changes that suggest more punitive and less compassionate public policies, it would seem that there is no incentive for HIV/AIDS and aging networks to work together. However, the clients of these two networks share many common experiences, such as stigmatization, isolation, and discrimination. Professionals from both arenas display tremendous commitment and dedication to their clients and recognize this professional integrity and dedication in one another. Bound by these common experiences, HIV/AIDS and aging professionals also recognize that their ability to serve clients, individually and collectively, will be enhanced as they reach across traditional program boundaries to tap the knowledge, perspective, and experience of professionals and advocates from aging services on the one hand and HIV/AIDS service arenas on the other.

REFERENCES

Allers, C. T. (1990). AIDS and the older adult. *The Gerontologist, 30*, 405–407.

Fleishman, J. A., Mor, V., Piette, J. D., & Allen, S. M. (1992). Organizing AIDS service consortia: Lead agency identity and consortium cohesion. *Social Service Review, 66*, 547–570.

Kern, S. (1989). AIDS education in longterm-care facilities. *Generations, XIII*(4), 64–66.

Lloyd, G. (1989). AIDS and elders: Advocacy, activism and coalitions. *Generations, XIII*(4), 32–35.

Nazon, M. (1992, May). *HIV/AIDS and Aging Task Force*. Paper presented at the 42nd Annual Conference of the National Council on Aging, Washington, DC.

Nazon, M. (1993, November). *HIV/AIDS and Aging Networks*. Paper presented at the 46th Annual Meeting of the Gerontological Society of America, New Orleans, LA.

Stall, R., & Catania, J. (1994). AIDS risk behaviors among late middle-aged and elderly Americans. *Archives of Internal Medicine, 154*, 57–63.

Stuen, C. (1990). Community organization, social planning and empowerment strategies. In A. Monk (Ed.), *Handbook of Gerontological Services*, 2nd ed. (pp. 168–192). New York: Columbia University Press.

Chapter 11

Voices

Dorothy E. Hickey

The stories of women and men who are aging with HIV/AIDS and the agencies that provide services to them offer a special dimension in understanding both the disease and its effect on individuals and groups. To hear these voices, telephone interviews were conducted by the author during the spring of 1995. An agency–organization interview format was structured to gather information about each group and the exclusive services it offers to women and men with HIV/AIDS who are over the age of 50. Information about staffing, funding, achievements, and future goals of the agency or organization, as well as about why, how, and when each of them decided to address HIV/AIDS in the over-50 population, was collected. The intent was to document the work of agencies throughout the United States and to explore models that could provide a resource or guide for other groups interested in offering similar services in their community.

The format used in facilitating the telephone interview with an agency–organization contact consisted of the following open-ended items: name, address, telephone number, name of contact, general and HIV/AIDS-specific purposes, motivations for addressing HIV/AIDS and the older person, methodology for addressing HIV/AIDS and the older person, length of time existing, funding source, number and professional preparation of paid staff, number and type of volunteers, achievements over the past 2 years, and goals for the next 2 years. In addition, the contact person was asked to submit a sample of an HIV/AIDS and aging publication that he or she used and to provide the names of other agencies or organizations addressing HIV/AIDS and aging. On completion of the agency–organization interview, the contact was asked to refer the author to individual(s) with HIV/AIDS who were more than 50 years of age and whom

---

Individual contributors: Allyn Gibson, Bill, Jane, Patrick Daniels, Sam, Sidney Morris, and the members of the Friends of Patrick.

they thought would agree to a telephone interview. (An overview of the questions used in the individual interviews were reviewed with the contact person). The agency–organization contact person made the initial contact with the older person with HIV/AIDS and then informed the author of their name, telephone number, and the best time to call. All of the older individuals with HIV/AIDS who were recommended by a contact person agreed to the telephone interview. In addition, two interview forms were completed anonymously by members of the Mt. Sinai group Friends of Patrick (see chapter 5).

In the case of an agency–organization, this method sometimes led to the identification of another agency–organization. More often the referred agency–organization served individuals over 50 with HIV/AIDS but did not offer a program specifically designed for their needs. Local AIDS hotlines were used to complete fragmentary information on referrals and to track potential leads, but these were not any more successful. Despite statistics acknowledging an aging population living with HIV/AIDS who have unique needs, there is still a striking lack of specially focused programs available to address this target group. Contacts of eight provider agencies–organizations from four areas (California, New Jersey, New York, and the District of Columbia) were interviewed. All but two of the individuals interviewed were referred from these providers. In designing the format for the individual interview, open-ended questions were constructed to facilitate a dialogue with a focus on their feelings. The format of the individual interview consisted of eliciting identifying information (name, address, telephone number, age, ethnicity, gender) and then, after saying "Let me tell you more about the things it would be helpful for you to share," the following open-ended questions:

- Would you like to start or for me to ask questions?
- How do you think you contracted HIV/AIDS?
- How do you feel about having HIV/AIDS?
- What as an older person has it meant for you to be HIV-positive?
- What difference do you think there is for you and a younger person with HIV/AIDS?
- How do you feel about your contacts with the health care system?
- Could you speak about the supports or lack of them you have experienced?
- Do you think you would have had the same response if you had cancer?
- Who has been assisting in your care?
- Do you have a message for the reader?

Individuals were offered the option of being identified by name if they chose. Six individuals were interviewed.

THEMES THAT EMERGED FROM AGENCY–
ORGANIZATION AND INDIVIDUAL INTERVIEWS

A number of themes surfaced from these interviews. Agencies–organizations servicing people over 50 with HIV/AIDS were developed within or under the leadership of established agencies–organizations; did not have special funding; offered group activities that focused on increased awareness, education, and support; had been formed in the past 5 years (most were only 2 years old); and depended on the skills, creativity, and commitment of the professionals who helped to develop them in response to an observed need. Individuals were found to be generous and open about their lives and how they became infected with HIV; most believed that they knew how they were infected; were eloquent in expressing personal philosophies (which included "time goes by and you live," "if it has to come, it has to come, I've had a lot of things in life others haven't," and "AIDS changed my life for the better"); were sensitive to the shortening of life span of younger people who were living with and dying from HIV/AIDS whom they had met, but were also aware of their own needs for separate services; were having difficulties sharing their HIV/AIDS diagnosis with family and friends because of their age; were finding it easier to actually deal with or imagine how they would discuss it if they had cancer rather than HIV/AIDS; were finding that others did not see them as still being sexual (where did YOU get it? or some variation was voiced several times); and were concerned about the lack of information and action by some physicians for someone in their age group with HIV/AIDS.

Three particular themes of aging people with HIV/AIDS are addressed in more detail. These include the impact of another loss along with those generally associated with the aging process, the lack of an understanding support group, and the response of others to the possibility of sexual activity at their age.

INTERVIEWS WITH OLDER PEOPLE
WITH HIV/AIDS

Patrick, a 58-year-old gay man from the "buckle on the Bible Belt" who contracted the virus through male–male sexual activity, was eloquent when he spoke. "I'm confronted with being four separate minorities: being gay, having AIDS, being blind, and aging." Growing up in rural America in the closet, "being a criminal, . . . my previous life prepared me to survive AIDS." He continued, "There is more meaning, focus, and direction in my life than before." He spoke of not having friends or family, "but people who work with me." He cannot see to write down appointments (he has two to four health-related ones a week) or remember ("vision supplies memory"). He has home care services, but one person sent to him could not read.

Patrick noted that he has outlived 12 separate support groups; "they don't support me, they're depressed, I'm not—I'm heroic, I'm dynamite, almost nobody like me." Some support services "can't deal with people my age or with long-term survivors. Many feel it's not normal and can't deal with the tension your existence brings up, they look at you like a production of *Oedipus Rex*." He felt his support comes from other older gay men. He expressed a feeling that older persons with AIDS have to be creative; "these are not afflictions but opportunities." As a member of the Advisory Council to the New York State Commission for the Blind, he has found a niche where he "can serve as a long-term survivor."

Sam, a 70-year-old, "traditional Jewish" heterosexual man, had bypass surgery in 1980, a stroke with visual impairment, and surgery for a malignant growth in 1993. He was "90% sure he was infected as a result of a transfusion." At first he "tried not to think" or felt that he would "go nuts." Thinking he would "be gone in a week or two," he wrote a letter for his wife to find after he died. Now despite arthritic pain, difficulty walking, fatigue, and depression, he has tried to go out daily for a walk and wishes he could just go out to a lounge and listen to jazz with his wife. He expressed his deep love for her and his fear of infecting her (she has tested negative twice). His wife "watches the toothpaste and towels" and will not permit sex or a kiss. He is working on a book of stories, which were told to him by his mother, to leave to his grandchildren, whom he does not see. "Unable to handle a group," Sam has received individual counseling and is taking an antidepressant medication. He still feels that he can handle his situation better than could a younger person.

Several of the respondents commented on the lack of a support group. A 72-year-old Black woman wrote, "I came to the group; that has been a support. Family is fine but they don't talk about it." She said that she was not sure how she had acquired the virus and did not know she had it until she got sick and the doctor told her she had HIV/AIDS.

Jane, a 55-year-old Irish American heterosexual woman and former secretary, contracted the virus during her first year of sobriety during sexual intimacy with a man she found out was using drugs. She had difficulty in finding people her age to relate to after receiving the result of an anonymous HIV test that she took after the deaths of several good Alcoholics Anonymous (AA) friends. She gained confidence in relating to others as she participated in speaking at 12-step meetings. While giving a presentation on HIV/AIDS to 12th graders, she recalled a youngster who asked her, "What are you doing here? You look like someone's mother." Jane's mother died when she was 4 years of age, her father died 30 years ago, and she has no siblings. She considered herself fortunate to now be living in secure housing managed by a local charity. Another support came from her relationship with her therapist in addition to her continued participation in AA. "I'm better now in speaking up."

Sidney, a 65-year-old Jewish man who identified himself as "born gay," has been a writer and activist. He had one lover for 10 years and another, who died in 1988, for 33 years. He now has lesions in his mouth related to HIV and owing to the progression of the illness has chronic diarrhea.

> Aging is no place for sissies. . . . It becomes a medical way of life, and AIDS is an extra burden. . . . Some people think you just come down with it; I've been struggling for years. . . . No one expected me to be around so long. . . . You have no immune backup, if you were just an elderly man you may lose your teeth.

In a prior support group, he was 20 to 30 years older than the other members. "When they would come to me they would say, 'Why should we listen to him, he's an old man.'" Having grown up with five sisters, he described himself as "a product of the '30's, life incomplete without mom in it." With lovers, he felt he always had someone next to him. He has found support in home visits from his therapist and from a warm, giving "angel" (volunteer) sent by the Actor's Fund until the latter's recent death. During a follow-up phone call, Sidney said that he is now in a new support group where he "feels useful and appreciated by the younger men."

Questions about differences older individuals felt between themselves and others who were younger and living with HIV/AIDS, their experiences with the health care system, and whether they thought that they would have had a different response if they had had a diagnosis of cancer rather than HIV/AIDS elicited a variety of responses.

A few clients felt that their contact with the health care system was good. Sam said he felt that he "was well treated in the hospital, no problems." The two anonymous respondents wrote that the system was good; however, neither of them noted that they had had an opportunistic infection requiring hospitalization. Jane said that she had been seeing a wonderful doctor in the clinic monthly until she became annoyed because gradually the physician did not spend enough time with her. She then sought a nurse practitioner in the clinic whom she felt was "very good, as nice as the doctor," and has been seeing her every month. She had pneumonia a year ago that did not require hospitalization. HIV-infected for 5 years, she is careful about what she eats and uses massage and acupuncture as needed. She considered herself "truly blessed; a lot of people are worse."

Allyn, a 63-year-old man, "a White southern human being," suspects he was infected through male–male sex. Even though he had been using condoms, one man insisted on not using them. He does not know this person's HIV status, as he moved away from the area. Diagnosed by an oral surgeon in 1992 with candidiasis, he has been treated and is now in good health. His contact with the health care system has been primarily with his primary care doctor, in a health maintenance organization, after anonymous HIV testing. Initially, he was seen by an infectious disease doctor whom he felt did not have enough knowledge. He saw Allyn for a 20-minute examination, placed him on medications, and told him to return in a couple of months.

Bill, a 53-year-old White Irish–English man, was "pretty sure" male–male sex was the source of his infection. He tested positive in 1987 but has not experienced any symptoms. He felt that the health care system has done a poor job of informing people about HIV/AIDS. After being told the results of his anonymous test, he was given information that was difficult for him to retain. When his insurance lapsed (he was laid off from his job and he did not wish to reveal his HIV status), he was dropped by his doctor. The physician had diagnosed thrush, "but he didn't do anything, he didn't care." He found very few doctors wanted HIV-positive (HIV+) patients and considered himself "lucky" that he found a clinic doctor who would take him on. He said he "cringes" when people say positive things about the health care system. He now sits on a primary care panel as a consumer and feels that with the increase in HMOs that there is a movement to "get rid of sick people." He has been going to a support group at a local mental health center for gay men and lesbians with HIV. Bill felt "the facilitators make a difference, that it is important to know there are others who have been there, this is not a death sentence. You can live." In his community, there is a hospice and assisted-living facility for HIV+ people. "It is very expensive, and federal guidelines only allow residency when you are practically homeless."

Patrick said he felt like an authority, "surviving 6 years of this stinking disease." It took him 5 years to find his present doctor at a local hospital. "Some doctors do research and disappear." Presently, he receives weekly visits from a nurse and a social worker, whom he feels that he "energizes." He felt he is deteriorating physically and his energy level is slowing. At first, he looked at life in 3-month increments but now looks at it year by year. "Another 5 years would be fabulous."

Sidney felt he had to educate his doctor, in particular, that people over age 60 do have sex. If he was hospitalized for any reason he knows, he said that he would be put on the AIDS unit. "People in the medical profession are prejudiced, they don't understand." When Sidney spoke of the difference in treatment he thought a person with cancer would receive as compared with that a person with HIV/AIDS would receive, he felt that blame is a key. "There is an added stress with HIV/AIDS, if the doctor will see you." The questions then are "Why did you get it?" and "Why did you go with more than one person?" He felt it is ironic because "people with AIDS get cancer—lymphoma."

Both Sam and Jane have had cancer. Sam said he had cancer and beat it, but "a contagious disease is stigmatizing." Jane was diagnosed with breast cancer the same week that she was told her HIV+ test result. "It was easy for me to tell people about the cancer but not HIV. I'm closed-mouthed about it, a private person. I only tell others what I want them to know." She told a close friend only about the cancer.

When asked if there was a difference between him and a younger person with an HIV/AIDS diagnosis, Bill said he has seen young people die and feels fortunate to be alive in his 50s. He has never felt "why me?" or been angry. "It's heartbreaking to see the deterioration of those in their 20s in the support group." He is divorced and has two sons.

Sidney said, "We live in a youth-oriented society across the board." Of the 12 young men he has been in contact with, none are left. Patrick expressed sadness for younger men: "If they lose their job they can't survive." He felt that he now has time to explore the things he loves. "Younger people don't realize their lives have been given back, you can't do anything when you are dead."

Allyn felt that as a college professor he has had an opportunity to use himself as a role model. In his professional practice, he can share his experience. "Younger people feel they have so many years ahead of them and go over the edge with a death threat." In coming out to his family, he experienced a freedom and release of pent-up energy. "I'm more at peace," he said.

Peace and sorrow were among the many feelings expressed by the people interviewed. This section closes with a few additional expressions of feelings voiced during these conversations. "Not happy . . . but what can I do? When I first found out I wanted to cry but I can't cry, I want[ed] to pray but I couldn't pray. I'm very sad about it." "I didn't get sober to get sick." "I saw many die. It's a scourge. It's unfair."

INTERVIEWS WITH AGENCY REPRESENTATIVES

Programs offered by agencies–organizations specifically targeted at people over 50 years of age with HIV/AIDS are divided into three categories; however, many offer services in more than one area. These groupings are education, peer support groups, and health services. A synopsis of each program, why each agency–

organization chose to address the need for service to individuals or groups who are over 50 years of age with HIV/AIDS, staffing patterns, funding, and achievements and goals of their program are presented. Contact with the individuals named for each entry is facilitated with the listing given in appendix D.

Agencies with education as their primary focus are the Coalition on AIDS in Passaic County (CAPCO) in New Jersey; Stop AIDS in California, and the American Association of Retired Persons (AARP) in Washington, DC.

CAPCO, as discussed earlier in this book (chapter 10), is a not-for-profit organization consisting of 45 member groups and individuals who are both providers and consumers. Their mission is to promote health education, prevention, and diagnostic services for HIV-infected persons. This is accomplished through networking and training opportunities for members and by providing recommendations to governmental bodies to assist in policy planning. The organization identified a need for testing and counseling services for people over age 50. Carol De Graw, the executive director of CAPCO, who is joint chairperson of this program with Daphne Joslin from William Paterson College, told the story of a woman in her 50s being refused testing despite perceived risk and unexplained symptoms because her doctor felt she was too old. Working together, CAPCO and the Office on Aging brought a production of skits on HIV/AIDS to six senior nutrition sites in Paterson, New Jersey. These skits were developed by the members of the Mental Health Players of Passaic County along with the Mental Health Association. The focus was on older adult dating and caretaking for themselves and others. The response to the production has been mixed. One of the identified problems was that caretakers do not have the opportunity to get to nutrition sites. There are six to eight very active CAPCO volunteers and no funding for this project. A future goal is to prepare a video in which affected and infected people over 50 are interviewed, with a particular concern for elderly persons who are caring for grandchildren. They would then assist in having the video shown on cable stations, in churches, and in congregate meal programs (see chapter 10).

The general purpose of Stop AIDS is education for safer sex, according to volunteer Dr. Leonard Kooperman. Identifying the incidence of HIV/AIDS to be more than 10% in those over 50 years of age, his group was directed specifically to gay–bisexual people in this age group. The group meets once for 4 hours, and a range of topics are presented in order to clarify the attendees' understanding of safer sex. During the meeting, attendees tell their stories and the impact HIV has had on their life. There are referrals for testing, and a telephone call is made 3 weeks after the meeting to follow up with information or referrals as needed. The program has been in existence for 2.5 years and receives funding through a Centers for Disease Control and Prevention (CDC) grant.

Judy Fink, an AARP senior program specialist, identified a need to direct attention and services to a population already experiencing the losses of aging, through her knowledge of AARP's Widowed Persons Service. AARP, as discussed earlier in this book, is the nation's leading organization for people 50 and older. It serves their needs and interests through legislative advocacy, research, informative programs, and community services provided by a network of local chapters and experienced volunteers throughout the country. The organization also offers members a wide range of special membership benefits, including *Modern Maturity* magazine and the monthly *AARP Bulletin*. Initially, Ms. Fink set up a half-day seminar for interested staff and invited representatives from CDC, Whitman-Walker Clinic, and a group of parents of lesbians and gay men; the program was met with an enthusiastic response. Fifty people attended, and the program continues as a lunchtime learning experience to the present. A team of 2–10 people from AARP who found this an interest in their lives for different reasons have worked on a variety of projects. A report on midlife and older women and HIV/AIDS and a fact sheet are available from AARP. Currently, AARP is working with the Brookdale AIDS and Aging Task Force to produce a videotape. It has also been assisting the Elderly Health Screening in Waterbury, Connecticut, with a poster campaign to include older faces in HIV health screening material. Fink felt that "the face of AIDS has changed in the '90s and there is a need to raise the awareness of people of all ages through the media to dispel myths." For the past 4 years, this team has been working on projects by giving their lunch and free time. The AARP receives membership fees and has 501C funding. There are two programs in the category of peer support groups: Iris Center in California and Friends of Patrick in New York (see chapter 5). The Iris Center is an outpatient substance use and mental health counseling service for women that has been in existence since late 1970 and receives federal funding through the Ryan White Care Act and private donations. Linda Martin, a HIV recovery counselor, has been the facilitator of a group called Women Over 40 that has been in existence since the fall of 1994. The group was started when several women over 40 in a substance abuse recovery group identified a need to meet and discuss their concerns about being HIV+. Topics of interest that have been addressed include menopause, fears concerning opportunistic infections, interactions with adult children, and substance abuse. A group of three to six women (three over 50) meet weekly for 2 hours. Sessions start with a half-hour relaxation period followed by an exchange called "What's New and What's Good." Martin said, "The women have expressed a feeling of safety in this connection with women who have similar issues."

The Friends of Patrick support group "germinated" in January 1993, was submitted as a proposal to the administration of Mt. Sinai Medical Center in March 1993 after a frequently revised needs assessment and had its first session in June 1993, according to Barbara Kornhaber. Kornhaber, a needle stick nurse at the medical center, and Mary Ann Malone, a social worker in the AIDS Center, sat next to one another at an AIDS conference when they heard a speaker named Patrick, who impressed them with the need for a group for those his age. They tapped into the clinic roster and sent letters of introduction to potential group members. The cofacilitators found that everyone in the group had acquired HIV/AIDS as a result of sexual transmission and were embarrassed to tell their family that they were sexually active. The group meets every other week and provides members with an opportunity to socialize and speak of their fears and loneliness. A psychiatrist provides supervision to the two cofacilitators, who sometimes relieve each another. As staff members, they incorporate the group into their day's activities but on their own time. In the group, the cofacilitators help the members to deal with HIV infection, provide education, and assist them in incorporating this information (see chapter 5).

The last category, health services, is illustrated by the work of three programs: Jeffrey Goodman Special Care Clinic of the Los Angeles Gay and Lesbian Community Services Center in California, Elder Family Services in New York, and Senior Action in a Gay Environment (SAGE), also in New York. The mission of the Los Angeles Gay and Lesbian Community Services Center is to provide mental health, education, training, and legal services to the gay and lesbian community. Over the past 3 years, the Jeffrey Goodman Special Care Clinic, a full-service primary care clinic located at the center, has identified an increasing number of clients over 50 in their population. They identified the names of 110 people in this age group from their census of 1,500. In addition, they found that 10% of the total census was over 50 and 2.5% were over 60. Joni Lavick, the clinical coordinator, told the author in an interview that they were having difficulties in groups the clinic offered because the other participants were so young. More than 3 years ago, a weekly psychosocial group began with 6 people. To date, 90 people have been participants in the educational and therapeutic sessions. Many ethnic groups are represented, along with gay men and heterosexual men and women. Some of the members have been consistent over the years, and others have had an on-and-off attendance. The clinic is staffed by 50 full-time and 15 part-time professionals, including a medical director, psychiatrists, registered nurses, and psychologists. Funding is from the Ryan White Care Act, organizational funds, private donations, and a share of center fundraising.

Karen Solomon, a social worker at Elder Family Services, spoke of the services this agency has been offering to those over age 50 since 1989. These include geriatric case management and guardianship for the adult population, as well as mental health services for those with the dual diagnosis of mental illness and chemical abuse. The staff of three full-time social workers—two with a geriatric background and one with an AIDS background—a part-time psychologist, and a psychiatrist see clients in the community and the hospital. After being approached by the Department of Mental Health in the fall of 1992, they set up the first HIV/AIDS services specifically for older adults. Elder Family Services staff work with affected homosexual, bisexual, and heterosexual women and men, including those infected through blood transfusion and substance users. Support groups are being added to the case management, which is now provided to 20–30 people. They also do outreach and education to older adults regarding AIDS. Solomon said people are still surprised and ask, "That's an issue?" when an elderly client is diagnosed with HIV/AIDS.

SAGE offers social services to gay and lesbian elderly persons (see chapter 6). According to Greg Anderson, former supervisor of individual services, SAGE has been in existence since 1978, offering comprehensive mental services, case management, support, and bereavement and caregivers groups. Through the AIDS and the Elderly program, which began in July 1989, those over age 50 living with HIV/AIDS are offered these services. In addition, SAGE offers public education on HIV/AIDS. Funding sources change yearly and presently include Ryan White for specific projects, Broadway Cares, and small grants (difficult to obtain) from the New York City Department of Health. The staff of SAGE consists of seven people—including two social workers, an administrator, a development director, and clerical staff—and 300 volunteers. The agency's achievements include raising the awareness of the gay–lesbian community, providing services to more than 200 individual people, providing public education, and a training program with the Burden Center on Aging. The latter is specifically for providers, offering them an opportunity to increase their skills in identifying, connecting with, and serving the gay–lesbian elderly. Goals for the future involve an expansion to a more comprehensive mental health model providing linkage and psychiatric services through the Ryan White Treatment Center.

All of these agencies–organizations that are recognizing the needs particular to this underserved and frequently unidentified population plan on continuing the same services, and many are expanding their projects in new directions. They are interested in sharing their history, organization, programs, achievements, and goals and were generous in giving their time for the interviews. Many of them also assisted in expediting contacts with clients. The author would also like to express her appreciation to Nathan Linsk of the University of Illinois, who was especially helpful in sharing his contacts and resources.

The final question that the author asked of all the persons with HIV/AIDS whom she interviewed was "Do you have a message for the reader?" These are some of the replies, the voices of those aging with HIV/AIDS: "Tell them to be careful." "If you are HIV+, be as positive as possible. Love yourself and trust God. Know that miracles happen." "If the reader is not HIV+, encourage them to be as knowledgeable as possible about its transmission, be accepting of those who are, and become involved as a volunteer." "Reevaluate your life, make changes." "AIDS represents a subtraction in people's live. You must help them find a way to compensate for the loss." "Some people think you just come down with it; I've been struggling for years. It's important to understand that inside every gay, aged person with a terminal disease may be a 7-year-old child [who] needs to be hugged too."

Appendix A

1993 Revised Classification System for HIV Infection and Expanded AIDS Surveillance Case Definition for Adolescents and Adults

CD4+ T-cell categories	Clinical categories		
	A: asymptomatic, acute (primary) HIV, or PGL[a]	B: symptomatic, not A or C conditions	C: AIDS-indicator conditions[b]
1. ≥500/μL	A1	B1	C1[c]
2. 200–499/μL	A2	B2	C2[c]
3. <200/μL (AIDS-indicator T-cell count)	A3[c]	B3[c]	C3[c]

[a]PGL = persistent generalized lymphadenopathy. Clinical Category A includes acute (primary) HIV infection.

[b]See the list of conditions on the following page.

[c]These illustrate the expanded AIDS surveillance case definition. Persons with AIDS-indicator conditions (Category C) as well as those with CD4+ T-lymphocyte counts less than 200/μL (Categories A3 and B3) will be reportable as AIDS cases in the United States and its territories effective January 1, 1993.

List of Conditions in the 1993 AIDS Surveillance Case Definition

Candidiasis of bronchi, trachea, or lungs
Candidiasis, esophageal
Cervical cancer, invasive[a]
Coccidioidomycosis, disseminated or extrapulmonary
Cryptococcosis, extrapulmonary
Cryptosporidiosis, chronic intestinal (>1 month duration)
Cytomegalovirus disease (other than liver, spleen, or nodes)
Cytomegalovirus retinitis (with loss of vision)
HIV encephalopathy
Herpes simplex (chronic ulcer[s]; >1 month duration) or bronchitis, pneumonitis, or
  esophagitis
Histoplasmosis, disseminated or extrapulmonary
Isosporiasis, chronic intestinal (>1 month duration)
Kaposi's sarcoma
Lymphoma, Burkitt's (or equivalent term)
Lymphoma, immunoblastic (or equivalent term)
Lymphoma, primary in brain
Mycobacterium avium complex or *M. kansasii*, disseminated or extrapulmonary
Mycobacterium tuberculosis, any site (pulmonary[a] or extrapulmonary)
Mycobacterium, other species or unidentified species, disseminated or extrapulmonary
Pneumocystis carinii pneumonia
Pneumonia, recurrent[a]
Progressive multifocal leukoencephalopathy
Salmonella septicemia, recurrent
Toxoplasmosis of brain
Wasting syndrome due to HIV

[a]These were added in 1993 expansion of the AIDS surveillance case definition.

EQUIVALENCES FOR CD4+ T-LYMPHOCYTE COUNT AND PERCENTAGE OF TOTAL LYMPHOCYTES

Compared with the absolute CD4+ T-lymphocyte count, the percentage of CD4+ T cells of total lymphocytes (or CD4+ percentage) is less subject to variation on repeated measurements. However, data correlating natural history of HIV infection with the CD4+ percentage have not been as consistently available as data on absolute CD4+ T-lymphocyte counts. Therefore, the revised classification system emphasizes the use of CD4+ T-lymphocyte counts but allows for the use of CD4+ percentages.

Definitive Diagnostic Methods for Diseases Indicative of AIDS

Disease	Diagnostic methods

Cryptosporidiosis
Isosporiasis
Kaposi's sarcoma
Lymphoma
Pneumocystis carinii
   pneumonia
Progressive multifocal
   leukoencephalopathy
Toxoplasmosis
Cervical cancer
	Microscopy (histology or cytology)

Candidiasis	Gross inspection by endoscopy or autopsy or by microscopy (histology or cytology) on a specimen obtained directly from the tissues affected (including scrapings from the mucosal surface), not from a culture.
Coccidioidomycosis Cryptococcosis Cytomegalovirus Herpes simplex virus Histoplasmosis Other mycobacteriosis	Microscopy (histology or cytology), culture, or detection of antigen in a specimen obtained directly from the tissues affected or a fluid from those tissues.
Salmonellosis Other bacterial infection Tuberculosis	Culture.
HIV encephalopathy (dementia)	Clinical findings of disabling cognitive or motor dysfunction interfering with occupation or activities of daily living, progressing over weeks to months, in the absence of a concurrent illness or condition other than HIV infection that could explain the findings. Methods to rule out such concurrent illness and conditions must include cerebrospinal fluid examination and either brain imaging (computed tomography or magnetic resonance) or autopsy.
HIV wasting syndrome	Findings of profound involuntary weight loss >10% of baseline body weight plus either chronic diarrhea (at least two loose stools per day for >30 days) or chronic weakness and documented fever (for >30 days, intermittent or constant) in the absence of a concurrent illness or condition other than HIV infection that could explain the findings (e.g., cancer, tuberculosis, cryptosporidiosis, or other specific enteritis).

Definitive Diagnostic Methods for Diseases Indicative of AIDS (*Continued*)

Disease	Diagnostic methods
Pneumonia, recurrent	Recurrent (more than one episode in a 1-year period) acute (new X-ray evidence not present earlier) pneumonia diagnosed by both (a) culture or other organism-specific diagnostic method of material obtained from a clinically reliable source of a pathogen that typically causes pneumonia (other than *Pneumocystis carinii* or *M. tuberculosis*) and (b) radiologic evidence of pneumonia; cases that do not have laboratory confirmation of a causative organism for one of the episodes of pneumonia will be considered to be presumptively diagnosed.

**Suggested Guidelines for Presumptive Diagnosis
of Diseases Indicative of AIDS**

Disease	Presumptive criteria
Candidiasis of esophagus	Recent onset of retrosternal pain on swallowing. Oral candidiasis diagnosed by the gross appearance of white patches or plaques on an erythematous base or by the microscopic appearance of fungal mycelial filaments in an uncultured specimen scraped from the oral mucosa.
Cytomegalovirus retinitis	A characteristic appearance on serial retinitis ophthalmoscopic examinations (e.g., discrete patches of retinal whitening with distinct borders, spreading in a centrifugal manner, following blood vessels, progressing over several months, frequently associated with retinal vasculitis, hemorrhage, and necrosis). Resolution of active disease leaves retinal scarring and atrophy with retinal pigment epithelial mottling. Mycobacteriosis microscopy of a specimen from stool or normally sterile body fluids or tissue from a site other than lungs, skin, or cervical or hilar lymph nodes, showing acid-fast bacilli of a species not identified by culture.
Kaposi's sarcoma	A characteristic gross appearance of an erythematous or violaceous plaquelike lesion on skin or mucous membrane. (Note: Presumptive diagnosis of Kaposi's sarcoma should not be made by clinicians who have seen few cases of it.)

**Suggested Guidelines for Presumptive Diagnosis
of Diseases Indicative of AIDS (*Continued*)**

Disease	Presumptive criteria
Pneumocystis carinii pneumonia	A history of dyspnea on exertion or nonproductive cough of recent onset (within the past 3 months), chest X-ray evidence of diffuse bilateral interstitial infiltrates or gallium scan evidence of diffuse bilateral pulmonary disease, arterial blood gas analysis showing an arterial pO_2 of <70 mm Hg or a low respiratory diffusing capacity (<80% of predicted values) or an increase in the alveolar–arterial oxygen tension gradient, and no evidence of a bacterial pneumonia.
Pneumonia, recurrent	Recurrent (more than one episode in a 1-year recurrent period), acute (new symptoms, signs, or X-ray evidence not present earlier) pneumonia diagnosed on clinical or radiologic grounds by the patient's physician
Toxoplasmosis	Recent onset of a focal necrologic abnormality consistent with intracranial disease or a reduced level of consciousness, brain-imaging evidence of a lesion having a mass effect (on computed tomography or nuclear magnetic resonance) or the radiographic appearance of which is enhanced by injection of contrast medium, and serum antibody to toxoplasmosis or successful response to therapy for toxoplasmosis.
Tuberculosis, pulmonary	When bacteriologic confirmation is not available, pulmonary and other reports considered to be verified cases of pulmonary tuberculosis using criteria of the Division of Tuberculosis Elimination, National Center for Prevention Services, Centers for Disease Control. The criteria in use as of January 1, 1993, are available in Morbidity and Mortality Weekly Reports 1990;39 (RR-13):39–40.

Appendix B

States Prohibiting Sexual Orientation Discrimination and Additional Resource Information

---

The following states have statewide legislation prohibiting discrimination on the basis of sexual orientation: California, Connecticut, Hawaii, Massachusetts, New Jersey, and Wisconsin. The District of Columbia also has such legislation.

The scope of the protection provided by these laws varies from state to state. For more information, check whether a state has an executive order that protects government employees. Also check whether a local civil rights or nondiscrimination ordinance may exist.

RESOURCES

Choice in Dying
250 W. 57th St.
New York, NY 10019

National Academy
  of Elder Law Attorneys
655 Alvernon St.
Suite 108
Tucson, AZ 85711

Brookdale Center on Aging
Institute on Law and Rights of Older Adults
425 E. 25th Street
New York, NY 10010

National Health Lawyers Association
1120 Connecticut Ave., NW
Washington, DC 20036-3902

Appendix C

Disposal Tips for Home Health Care

You can help prevent injury, illness, and pollution by following these simple steps when disposing of sharp objects and contaminated materials used in administering health care in the home: Needles, syringes, lancets, and other sharp objects should be placed in a hard plastic or metal container with a screw-on or tightly secured lid. A coffee can will do, but the plastic lid should be reinforced with heavy-duty tape. Do not put sharp objects in any container that will be recycled or returned to a store. Do not use glass or clear plastic containers. Finally, make sure that containers with sharp objects are kept out of the reach of young children.

It is also recommended that soiled bandages, disposable sheets, and medical gloves be placed in securely fastened plastic bags before putting them in the garbage can with other trash.

From the United States Environmental Protection Agency, 530-SW-90-014B, January 1990.

Appendix D

Resources for Grandparents

California Coalition for Grandparents Parenting Grandchildren
University of California
2420 Bowditch St.
Berkeley, CA 94720
510-643-7538
Contact: Priscilla Enriquez

California Coalition of Grandparent and Relative Caregivers
GOLD
700 N. Johnson Ave., #0
El Cajon, CA 92020
619-477-7349
Contact: Margie Davis
or
4701 San Leandro St., #44
Oakland, CA 94601
510-535-1996
Contact: Ed Warren

Florida "Second Chance" Coalition
St. Petersburg Free Clinic, Inc.
863 Third Ave. North
St. Petersburg, FL 33701
813-821-1200
Contact: Jane Trocheck Walker

New York Committee for Kinship Family Care
Institute for Families and Children
200 Church St.
New York, NY 10013
212-233-5051
Contact: Pamela Jones

New York Grandcare
56 Bay St.
New York, NY 10301
718-981-9226
Contacts: Margaret Hammer and Margaret McDevitt

Harlem Hospital Program for Grandparent Caregivers
Harlem Hospital Center
Department of Child and Adolescent Psychiatry
506 Lennox Ave., 5K
New York, NY 10037
212-939-3129 or 212-939-3133
Contacts: Gloria Maldonado and Jacqueline Walker

Northwest Coalition of Grandparents
Tacoma-Pierce County Health Departments
3629 S. D St.
Tacoma, WA 98408
206-591-6490
Contact: Edith Owen

Children's Rights Coalition
P.O. Box 254
West Linn, OR 07068
800-440-KIDS or 503-288-3129
Contact: Sina Johnson

D.C. Kinship Care Coalition
Children's Hospital
Department of Social Work
111 Michigan Ave., NW
Washington, DC 20010
202-884-5214
Contact: Brenda Shepard-Vernon

Appendix E

Where Older Persons with HIV Disease Can Get Help and Additional Agencies and Organizations

The problem of AIDS in persons 50 and older has received little recognition. However, a few organizations now provide literature or services aimed specifically at older patients and their health care providers.

American Association of Retired Persons
601 E St. NW
Washington, DC 20049
202-434-2293
202-434-6474 (Fax)
Contact: Judy Fink

Publishes free fact sheet, "AIDS: A Multigenerational Crisis" (Stock No. D14941) that includes listings of referral services.

Senior Action in a Gay Environment (SAGE)
305 Seventh Ave.
New York, NY 10001
212-741-2247
212-366-1947 (Fax)
Contact: Arlene Kochman

Provides a variety of services to gay persons in their 50s or older. Also offers training, education, counseling, and therapy and is a source of information for physicians and hospitals. Operates chiefly in the area surrounding New York City (New York, New Jersey, and Connecticut).

Healthcare Education Associates
70 Campton Pl.
Laguna Niguel, CA 92677
714-240-2179

Publishes a training manual for use in discussion groups, *AIDS and Aging: What People Over 50 Need to Know. Leader's Guide* and *Participant's Workbook* are $13.95; workbook alone is $5.00.

HIV/AIDS in Aging Task Force
425 E. 25th St.
New York, NY 10010
212-481-7670 or 212-636-9484

Arranges conferences and educational seminars; participants include a variety of health and social service providers. Provides support for establishing task forces and seminars throughout the country.

National Institute on Aging
Public Information Office
Federal Bldg. 31 (Room 5C27)
Bethesda, MD 20892
301-496-1752

Publishes fact sheet, "Age Page: AIDS and Older Adults"; available as a fax transmission by calling 800-222-2225.

Elder Family Services
494 9th St.
Brooklyn, NY 11215
718-788-2461
718-788-8274 (Fax)
Contact: Joan Zimmerman

Iris Center
333 Valencia, Suite 222
San Francisco, CA 94103
415-864-2364
415-864-0116 (Fax)
Contact: Linda Martin

Jeffrey Goodman Special Care Clinic, Los Angeles
Gay/Lesbian Community Services Center
1625 N. Schnader Blvd.
Los Angeles, CA 90028
213-993-7521
213-993-7599 (Fax)
Contact: Joni Lavick

Mount Sinai Medical Center
1 Gustave Levy Plaza, Box 1009
New York, NY 10029
212-241-5911
Contact: Mary Ann Malone
212-831-1127 (AIDS Center Fax)

Stop AIDS
Golden Gate University
School of Public Service
536 Mission
San Francisco, CA 94105
415-442-7873
Contact: Leonard Kooperman

The Coalition on AIDS in Passaic County, Inc.
175 Market St., Room 207
Paterson, NJ 07505
201-742-6742
201-742-6750 (Fax)
Contact: Carol De Graw

Index

Printed in the United States
by Baker & Taylor Publisher Services